The Ventricle of Memory

Personal Recollections of Some Neurologists

The Ventricle of Memory
Personal Recollections of Some Neurologists

Macdonald Critchley, M.D.

Raven Press New York

Raven Press, Ltd., 1185 Avenue of the Americas, New York, New York 10036

Library of Congress Cataloging-in-Publication Data

Critchley, Macdonald.
    The ventricle of memory.

    Includes bibliographical references.
    1. Neurologists—Biography. I. Title. [DNLM: 1.
Neurology—biography. WZ 112.5.N4 C934v]
RC339.5.C75 1990   616.8′092′2   89-11003
ISBN 0-88167-599-7

The material contained in this volume was submitted as previously unpublished material, except in the instances in which credit has been given to the source from which some of the illustrative material was derived.

9 8 7 6 5 4 3 2 1

Preface

According to Peter Quennell, "Biography is a rewarding branch of literature. One relives the past, moves through the crowded scenes of an unfamiliar social period, makes odd friends, is told fantastic stories . . ." He also said, "To be remembered, talked over, even perhaps sometimes laughed at, is surely the only tribute that the dead require."

I am not quite old enough to have met Hughlings Jackson, Gowers, Charcot, Edinger or Pierre Marie—those giants of neurology—but my teachers and senior colleagues knew them well. I met Ferrier, Henry Head, Pavlov, Nonne, Barney Sachs, Charles Dana and T. H. Weisenburg; and have conversed with Bonhoeffer, Bumke, André-Thomas and Egas Moniz. But the lives of all these notable figures have been well documented.

No mention has been made here of James Collier, Gordon Holmes or Kinnier Wilson, all of whom were my teachers, colleagues and friends, because I have already written about them.

However, there were other neurological friends, now departed, who have not yet been accorded such a degree of written attention despite the achievements and prestige they acquired. One or two may, in time, be forgotten. I have not attempted to cover the bare facts of their careers, nor to write full biographies. I wanted to write only my impressions of them as their lives crossed mine. All were my friends; all I hold in high esteem.

When I use the word *neurologist* in these pages it applies in its widest sense, in that it indicates those who chose to study the brain and the nervous system in all its aspects. Three of my sketches are of neurosurgeons, and a few would probably be considered neuropsychiatrists or neuropsychologists today.

What I had in mind was to rummage in my cache of memories and bring up a medley of people whom I miss and whose contributions to neurology I earnestly hope will survive.

"Egregious and arcane science of physic, of your urbanity, exasperate not yourselves against me for making this volume."

Macdonald Critchley

Nether Stowey, Somerset
1989

For Eileen
"The ocean to the river of my thoughts"

Acknowledgments

Several colleagues have been most helpful in my quest for information. In particular, I am in debt to the generous assistance afforded by Dr. Robert Joynt of Rochester, New York; Dr. Leon Whitsell of San Francisco; and Professor Michael Shepherd of the Institute of Psychiatry, London. Others who have kindly helped me are Professor Refsum and Professor Per Dietrichsen of Oslo; Professor George Bruyn of Leiden; Professor John H. Tyrer of Brisbane; and Professor James Lance of Sydney. Also, Professor Pichot of Paris.

To the staff of many medical libraries I extend my grateful thanks. Particular recognition is due to Mrs. Beryl Bailey of the

Rockefeller Library at the Institute of Neurology, London; and to Mrs. Lucretia McClure, Librarian to the School of Medicine, Dentistry and Nursing, Rochester, New York. Their enthusiastic help has been invaluable. The Librarians of the Royal College of Physicians, the Royal Society of Medicine, the London Hospital School of Medicine, the Royal Society, the Medical School of the University of Newcastle upon Tyne, have been most helpful. My particular appreciation is due to Mme. Pierrette Cassayre, the Conservateur of the Académie Nationale de Médecin.

Mrs. Sissel Cooper has kindly allowed me to quote several passages from her late husband's autobiography *The Vital Probe*, and she has also permitted me to reproduce a photograph of Dr. Irving Cooper. Mrs. Sara Bender has enabled me to include a photograph of her husband, Morris. Lady Butterfield of Cambridge was most generous in presenting me with a photograph of her father, Dr. Foster Kennedy, which I reproduce with her kind permission.

The Institute of Neurology and the Royal College of Physicians of London have courteously allowed me to replicate several of the photographs in the text. The Editor of the Journal of the Mount Sinai Hospital has been kind in allowing me to utilize the portrait of Dr. Israel Wechsler.

Edward Arnold kindly made prints for me of Drs. Alajouanine, Grewel and Luria which appeared originally in my *Aphasiology* and was published by them in 1970.

I am beholden to Mr. Peter Quennell and his publishers, Weidenfeld & Nicolson, for allowing me to quote two passages from *Customs and Character*. For permitting me to quote from Richard Llewellyn's *How Green Was My Valley*, I am indebted to the publishers Michael Joseph Ltd.

My wife, Eileen, has been unstinting in her encouragement. Her wise and sensitive criticisms on what I have written, have been invaluable, even vital. She also devoted many precious months to transcribing my scribble into longhand, so that I could revise the script before it was typed.

Contents

1886–1935
William J. Adie

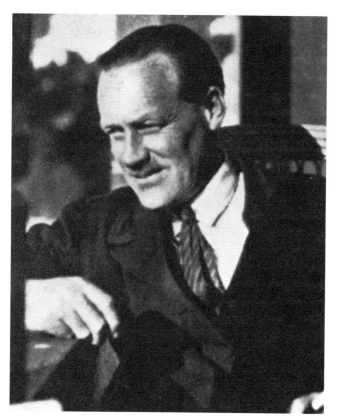

WILLIAM J. ADIE

Courtesy of the Institute of Neurology, London.

S ometimes, fortunately not often, Fate is incomprehensibly unkind. A few neurologists like E.G. Fearnsides, Hamilton Paterson, Paul Schilder, George Riddoch, Hughes Bennett, J.L. Birley and Charles Foix have died comparatively young men, full of academic promise, to the detriment of their discipline. William Adie was one of those whose loss I personally grieved, both as a friend and an outstanding clinician.

He was born in 1886 in Geelong, Victoria, Australia. After attending Flinders School in Geelong, he went to Scotland for his medical training. Like his senior, and more famed colleague Kinnier Wilson, he too attained his M.D. Edinburgh, with the added distinction of being a gold medallist.

He pursued postgraduate studies in Berlin and Munich, and became fluent in the German language. Adie never spoke to me of his student days in Germany, nor did he discuss his teachers. Presumably in Berlin he attended the clinics of Lewandowsky and Oppenheim at the Charité Hospital. Adie's mastery of the language enabled him to keep abreast with the neuropsychiatric literature of Germany and Austria, which, up to the Hitler hegemony, was prolific and conspicuous in quality.

In 1913, Adie was appointed House Physician to the National Hospital, Queen Square, about the same time as F.M.R. Walshe and J.L. Birley. William Gowers had recently retired and was in poor health. Hughlings Jackson had died two years before, but the influence of these two geniuses was pervasive and still felt by all who worked in that hospital.

With the advent of the first World War in August, 1914, Adie immediately joined the Army and was appointed Medical Officer to the Northamptonshire Regiment. He was at once sent to France. Participating in the retreat from Mons, he became one of the "old contemptibles". Later, and while still in the British Expeditionary Force, he was attached to the 7th General Hospital. Still later, he was made Consultant to the 2nd Army Centre for Head Injuries.

Three years after the war ended, he became an Assistant Physician to the National Hospital.

As I remember him in 1923, he was of medium height, slightly bronzed in complexion, with brown hair sleeked back, and with a clipped moustache. Had he been encountered in Aldershot, he would have been identified as a Brigade Major off duty. His voice, however, was mild, and he spoke with slow deliberation. Despite his obvious abilities and his considerable private practice, he was a friendly man, devoid of arrogance.

Adie soon established himself as a popular clinical neurologist. For a time he was on the consulting staff of The Royal Northern Hospital. This, however, was not a teaching hospital, and he resigned when he was appointed to Charing Cross Hospital, then sited close to Trafalgar Square. There he was junior to, though in no way overpowered by, the great Gordon Holmes. If Adie recognised any maestro among his older colleagues at Queen Square, it was that brilliant eccentric, James Collier. Adie was also invited to become a consulting neurologist to the Royal London Ophthalmic Hospital, better known as Moorfields.

At the National Hospital, Adie was held in high esteem, although there was mutual dislike between Kinnier Wilson and himself. The former always referred to the latter as "colleague Adie". Adie's rejoinder is unprintable.

Today, Adie is largely forgotten, but during his lifetime he was an inspiring teacher especially to postgraduates at Queen Square. Like the rest of us, he was a showman. He also indulged himself in that impressive art of rapid diagnosis. Unlike some other lightning operators, he delighted in explaining the perceptual and conceptual steps that he had invoked in reaching a diagnosis.

His students became familiar with the key to Adie's instant recognition of general paralysis of the insane—then a not uncommon disorder. The patient would present himself always with his wife in attendance. Invariably he had neglected to remove his cap. Asked "What is the matter?", the patient would turn to his wife for her to reply. But when the doctor insisted that the husband should answer, the patient, with trembling lips, would slur "n-n-n-neuraesthenia".

Occasionally, when there was little "teaching material" for him to demonstrate, Adie would reminisce. I remember him telling his class of students that late the previous evening, a doctor telephoned him about a puzzling case. Adie felt too weary to drive far into the suburbs, and asked whether he could discuss the case over the telephone. "My patient", said the doctor, "is a middle-aged lady previously in good health. This morning she complained that the whole of one side 'felt funny'. She could move her arm and leg but they tingled. It was the other side of the face, however, which 'felt different'. She had no pain but she was dizzy and nauseated. She was offered a cup of tea, but, as she moved the cup to her lips, she spilled the liquid. With help, she was able to drink, only to find some difficulty in swallowing. What could be the matter?". Still on the telephone, Adie replied, "Tell me, doctor, on which side is the smaller pupil?". The doctor answered, "The right, as a matter of fact." Adie replied, "Your patient has sustained a thrombosis of the right posterior inferior cerebellar artery. She will probably slowly but steadily improve."

On another occasion, a youngish woman came into Adie's clinic, saying that her legs were becoming more and more unsteady, and that her hands, too, were clumsy. She was becoming increasingly deaf in both ears, and of late she had been getting headaches. "Gentlemen," said Adie, "this is an example of von Recklinghausen's disease associated with bilateral acoustic neurofibromata. She has a cerebellar syndrome resulting from direct pressure. And, gentlemen, do you notice a couple of papules on her forehead and on her chin? And look—just at the cleavage of her blouse—there is a distinct café-au-lait patch."

There was one occasion, however, when Homer nodded, and I was taken off guard. A woman was seen by Adie in Out-Patients, and was diagnosed and demonstrated as a case of syringomyelia. She was admitted under Gordon Holmes. As his House Physician, I made detailed notes of the muscle-wasting and I prepared elaborate charts of her areas of thermanalgesia. The day came for Holmes to make rounds. He paused for a moment at the foot of the patient's bed, then swung round, grabbed me by the lapels of my jacket and ran me out of the ward. "What the blazes do you mean by admitting to my ward a case of leprosy?". Of course, his diagnosis was right. Incidentally, this was the only time I ever saw Holmes make a spot diagnosis.

Like Adie, I was becoming conversant with the German literature, thanks to the cooperation of my tutor. It was inevitable that Adie and I should read and be impressed by an important paper upon the *Greifreflex* published by Schuster and Pinéas of Berlin. Both Adie and I had patients with an odd one-sided grasping propensity. A fruitful collaboration followed, resulting in our paper entitled "Forced grasping and groping". We were able to confirm and also to elaborate the findings of Schuster and Pinéas, but we differed in their interpretation. They attributed the phenomenon to the basal ganglia. We invoked the frontal lobes, and this view subsequently proved to be correct. Correspondence with the German authors led to a close friendship between Schuster and myself.

The paper by Adie and me was published in *Brain* in 1927. It was followed by another communication on the same topic, praising us with faint damns. Obviously we had not been fully understood. As I have so frequently said, misinterpretation is often the fault of the writer rather than the reader. Boileau asserted that what is not crystal clear is not French. The critics were my good friends F.M.R. Walshe and Graeme Robertson. A five-minute colloquy would have settled the matter.

Adie is perhaps best remembered for his isolation of a clinical phenomenon comprising a symptomless myotonic type of reaction of the pupils coupled with an absence of tendon reflexes. Adie's syndrome, as it is usually called, is an inexplicable state of affairs. It often leads to the suspicion of tabes, though close scrutiny of the pupillary reaction reveals important differences from the Argyll Robertson phenomenon. It is observed far more often in women than in men, and frequently the pupillary anomaly is uniocular.

Unfortunately, Adie's papers upon this subject, which appeared in 1931 and 1932, provoked some ill-feeling. Adie was accused of ignoring a paper on the same topic written by Gordon Holmes in 1932, as well as an article by Gayer Morgan and C.P. Symonds. I am convinced that Adie was unaware of these papers; he protested this to me many times. Holmes himself made no complaint, as far as I know; it would not have been in his nature to feel aggrieved at not being quoted. Some other neurologists, however, were loud in their condemnation of Adie, hinting broadly at sheer plagiarism. Had Adie been following the British literature as closely as the German, he would not have erred. Today, one is more likely to refer to the Holmes-Adie syndrome.

Yet another of Adie's contributions to the literature proved to be an embarrassment. He had become deeply interested in narcolepsy, a condition described in 1880 by J.B.E. Gelineau. The original paper had secured scant attention but Adie's clinical acumen had unearthed a number of such cases, causing him to realise the complexity of the syndrome. The social hazards and mental distress engendered by the symptoms, were emphasized by Adie. By an odd coincidence, Kinnier Wilson had also become aware of this strange syndrome, and, quite independently, was collecting his own series of cases. Adie finished his paper first, and his comprehensive account of narcolepsy appeared in *Brain* in 1926; Wilson's article was not published until 1928, but he never forgave Adie. He rejected Adie's claim that narcolepsy was a disorder *sui generis,* asserting that the condition was symptomatic, the commonest cause being encephalitis. He preferred to speak of "the narcolepsies". In 1930 Adie published a further paper in *The Practitioner,* and restated that narcolepsy was indeed an idiopathic, isolated entity; he also emphasized that it was a not uncommon condition.

If questions of priority are to provoke such ill-feeling, it is as well to remember that in 1685 Thomas Willis described this syndrome in his *London Practice of Physicke.*

Yet another condition, earlier described by Meyer and also by Gelineau, appealed to Adie's interest in the unusual. The term "pyknolepsy" had been used to describe a paediatric syndrome of an exceptionally large number of *petit mal* attacks which eventually and permanently cease. The "cure" could not be ascribed to treatment, but came about spontaneously and mysteriously. Adie wrote a full account of this condition in 1924 (*Brain,* vol. 47). The syndrome failed to receive enthusiastic acceptance, and in retrospect it seems likely that pyknolepsy belongs to the no-man's land of neurology, being one of a number of mythical maladies of the nervous system.

In the period 1923–1935, there were few textbooks available to neurological students except, of course, Gowers' *Manual of Diseases of the Nervous System*—the Bible of Neurology. In 1922 Dr. Price, a London cardiologist, published a multi-author handbook of medicine. Diseases of the nervous system were delegated to James Collier, who immediately invited Adie to collaborate. The result was remarkably successful. Some students—myself included—would buy the book, tear out the pages devoted to neurology, tenderly bind them, and discard the rest of the volume. For many years, the Collier-Adie synergy was unrivalled. Today, bound copies of the torn-out pages are prized by medical bibliophiles.

Personally, I am grateful to Adie for some shrewd remarks he made to me. It was the duty of an Assistant Physician to the National Hospital to attend the Out-Patient Department twice a week. Teaching took place only in "A" room, being carried out by one of the Physicians in Charge of Out-Patients. The Assistant Physician sat alone in "B" room, his clientele comprising, for the most part, chronic epileptics. Medication would be prescribed, and issued at the hospital dispensary. The patient would return in one, two or three months' time to report progress and to receive a further supply of drugs.

Some doctors regarded these clinics as intolerably boring. Not so Adie. This experience, he told me, taught him to listen to the patient's comments. In that way he gained a deep understanding of the natural history of epilepsy, the vagaries of the fit-incidence, and the mental, physical and social concomitants of the malady.

When the time came for me to sit in "B" room, I was able to confirm to the full what Adie had said. By allowing each patient to ramble on unchecked, I stumbled upon such curiosities as reading epilepsy and musicogenic epilepsy.

Over and above all these hospital activities, Adie carried out a large and fashionable private practice. His consulting rooms were in Brook Street, Mayfair, just outside "pill-island", that is, the Wimpole Street–Harley Street enclave. His residence was in one of the elegant Nash terraces facing Regent's Park.

Never once during the 12 years I knew him and was the confidant of his many anxieties, did I enter his house. I was not alone. At that time before the second World War, hospitality was the rule, and house officers and junior colleagues were frequently invited to dine at home with their seniors, less often in a restaurant.

Adie was the victim of chronic ill-health, being constantly plagued by precordial pain. Nevertheless, he carried on.

It was sometime during the 1930s that the National Hospital was visited by that scholarly oddity Dr. Smith Ely Jelliffe. At that time he was advocating a strange holistic philosophy, being critical of conventional diagnostic labels. His views upon the aetiology of multiple sclerosis astonished us. We listened in subdued amazement. Shortly afterwards Adie said to me, "I was driving home one night, miserable and dead tired from seeing so many patients at the hospital and then at Brook Street. Suddenly I thought of Jelliffe, and I cried aloud 'Cheer up, Bill Adie, there's no such thing as a disease', and I threw back my head and laughed and laughed, and by the time I got home I felt almost alive."

The cracked pitcher goes once too often to the well, and it was in one of his many attacks of anginal pain that Adie died at the age of 49 on 17th March 1935. His wife and his two children survived him.

Looking back over Adie's life and works, I am reminded of W.S. Gilbert's lyric in *The Gondoliers:*

Talented, cultivated, under-rated,
Unaffected, undetected, well-connected.
Ever knowing, overflowing, easy going.

1890–1980
Théophile Alajouanine

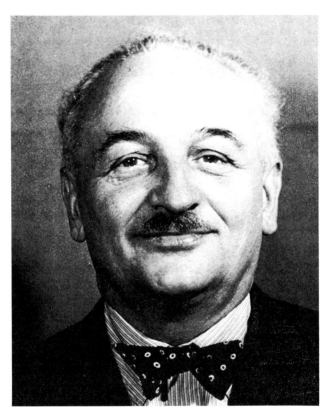

THEOPHILE ALAJOUANINE

My first meeting with Professor Alajouanine sticks firmly upon my flypaper memory. It was early in the Thirties, and George Riddoch had given me a letter of introduction to him. I preferred to present it to him in his clinic at the Bicêtre, rather than invade the privacy of his home.

The Bicêtre made me realise the great difference in the mode of dress adopted by French as opposed to British physicians. At the National Hospital, the consultants visited the wards in ordinary suits. Kinnier Wilson was an exception, for he preferred to wear a long white coat.

In France the practice is more elaborate. Thus, Alajouanine was wearing an enveloping surgical gown from chin to ankles, fastened at the back with tapes. Another tape was tied around his middle. Over the gown was an apron with two capacious pockets. A white cotton cap concealed his hair, or perhaps his baldness.

The Professor was busy studying a patient with footdrop. The victim, an insignificant little man in his 40s, with glasses and an untidy moustache, was retailing the history of his symptoms. He had happened to call in upon a widow of his acquaintance. One thing had led to another, and the widow had perched herself upon his lap. She was a heavily built lady and gradually her visitor's leg began to tingle. He did not like to complain, for he did not know her very well. When at last she got off, he found that his right foot was dead and useless and had remained so ever since.

Confronted with such a saga, and despite my ten years at Queen Square, I was a diagnostic innocent.

I must have expressed my wonder at such an unusual story,

for Alajouanine remarked "This is nothing out of the ordinary; it is a clear case of '*la paralysie des amoureux*'."

Thus began my lifelong respectful friendship with one who has been described as *le clinicien hors de pair*.

Théophile Alajouanine was born on 12th June 1890 in Verneix, a small village in the heart of France, where his father was a master locksmith. A paternal cousin, who was a priest, recognised the boy's high intelligence and arranged for him to be educated at a select Marist seminary at Moulins, the capital town of Allier. With consummate ease he passed into the University of Paris, selecting medicine as his goal. As an intern he gained the gold medal.

With the onset of the 1914 war, Alajouanine became a Battalion Medical Officer, served on the Somme and also at Verdun, being twice mentioned in *Despatches* and winning the *Croix de Guerre* with two citations. Then he was transferred to the Middle East, where he became neurologist to the hospital in Salonika. There he met an English nurse, whom he married.

When the war ended he was attached to the service of Dejerine and Pierre Marie at the Salpêtrière, where he met Charles Foix. The latter became Alajouanine's devoted friend, elder brother and master until his sudden death in 1927. Alajouanine never ceased to refer to this great man. When, in 1947, he was appointed to the Charcot Chair of Neurology, Alajouanine remarked in his opening address that had the blind Fates not stepped in, it would have been Foix and not himself who would be addressing the concouse and succeeding Charcot, Raymond, Brissaud, Dejerine, Pierre Marie and Guillain.

On his accession to the Charcot Chair, Alajouanine moved his service to the ancient and famed Salpêtrière. Originally a gunpowder factory, it had become in turn a refuge for down-and-outs, a penal institution for fallen women (among them Manon Lescaut), and an asylum for the insane—open to the public gaze. It was here the reformer Pinel had insisted that the wretched lunatics, chained and lying on straw, should be unshackled. Today, trees and gardens grow between grey buildings and possess a curious charm that was captured by Jean Delay (under the pen-name Jean Faurel), one-time Professor of Psychiatry, in his novello *La Cité Grise.*

In another piece, which he termed *Les Réposantes,* he wrote of the frail old ladies sitting on the benches warming their thin bodies in the sun. There they sat, most of them in silence but sometimes chatting of past glories as courtesans, or maybe just concièrges or housewives. Preserved intact within the compound was Charcot's library, with its gallery and bound volumes of his case-notes. Over his desk hung a framed photograph of Hughlings Jackson.

Many times since then have I lunched and dined with him and he with me in London. We talked together, occasionally argued, frequently chuckled.

From time to time, Alajouanine invited me to give talks to his students at the Salpêtrière. Once my subject was Alphonse Daudet's tabes, for I had discovered a copy of his diary in which he vividly described his symptoms. Alajouanine was fascinated, because I had turned up a literary fragment of which he had known nothing. Another time I lectured on speech iterations and I spoke of the "ting-a-ling" syndrome, so dubbed by me because of a British music hall song of that name. At the end of the lecture, Alajouanine asked for the slide showing the lyric of the song to be shown again. He then insisted upon my singing it to him, much to the students' amusement.

I came to realise that this little man, 10 inches shorter than me, with his perpetual roguish smile and forever rolling cigarettes, was not only a great neurologist but a man of considerable culture. His circle of friends comprised writers, painters and musicians; but, above all, he was a bibliophile. He collected books, not because of their antiquarian value or their scarcity, but in order to read them. His library was immense, and many of the volumes had dedications personally signed by the authors. He knew more about English literature than many British graduates. He was the only Frenchman I knew who was a subscriber to *The Times Literary Supplement.*

As a neurologist, Alajouanine was an all-rounder, not unlike C.P. Symonds but with a profound, absorbing interest in aphasia. It is not surprising that one who was so fascinated with language, French or English, would also be intrigued with the consequences of its dissolution.

He published one of the most successful short monographs on aphasia, comparable only with the bibelot written by Kinnier Wilson. Alajouanine was one of the first to realise the importance of phonetics in the investigation of aphasiacs. He has been called the first of the neurolinguists, a title which he disliked and which was not appropriate. He collaborated with a psychologist (Ombredane) and a linguist (Durand) in studying the articulatory defects in aphasiacs. They proffered the idea that aphasiacs underwent an articulatory disintegration that recapitulated the steps taken in childhood when learning to master the various phonemes. This was an attractive idea, but one which could not be substantiated when I sent a recording of the speech of one of my patients for analysis by Professor D.B. Fry of the Department of Phonetics of the University of London in 1959. Later, Alajouanine wrote a detailed monograph on the pathology of speech, in association with André Roch Lecours (now in Montreal).

Alajouanine interested himself deeply in the treatment of patients with disordered language, and thus inaugurated at the Salpêtrière the Centre du Langage, which is today known the world over.

One classic occasion was Alajouanine's lecture delivered before the Harveian Society of London and subsequently published in *Brain* in 1956. This was his study of "Artistic Realisation in Aphasia", in which he described the effect of a speech-loss upon the musical life of a composer, the writings of a famous French *littérateur,* and the work of a landscape painter. Although he did not reveal the identity of these patients, it is no secret that he was referring to Ravel, Valéry-Radaud and

Verniez respectively. In the case of the last-named, no falling-off could be detected in the quality of his work after he lost his speech. Alajouanine showed me two landscape paintings on the walls of his drawing-room, one painted by this artist before his aphasia and one after. "Which is which?," he asked me; I was unable to answer. According to at least one art critic, so Alajouanine said, there was a subtle betterment noticeable in the artist's brushwork after the stroke that had caused his aphasia. In Ravel's case, however, matters were different. He had been seen by other doctors, as fully discussed by Dr. Ronald Henson in his address published in *The British Medical Journal* on 4th June 1988.

One of Alajouanine's first appearances in print, with Professor Laignel-Lavastine, described a case of auditory agnosia. Laignel-Lavastine was destined to become a famed psychiatrist. It was he who was called upon to examine the notorious mass murderer of 1942–1943, Dr. Marcel Pétiot.

When I was President of the Harveian Society, I decided to give my Presidential address on a criminological topic. Highly topical was the extraordinary story of Dr. Pétiot. On my behalf, Alajouanine kindly exerted his influence with the French Minister of Justice, and I was allowed access to the complete dossier of the case in the *Préfecture de Police*.

Our mutual interest in aphasia led, in a roundabout fashion, to an event which was unforgettable.

While on holiday in France and motoring beyond Nîmes en route to Montpellier, I saw a signpost indicating that Sommières was close by. This had been the home of Dr. Marc Dax and his son, Dr. Gustave Dax. Dr. Marc Dax was believed to be the first to realise that language was a function more of the left than the right half of the brain. I made a detour and found Sommières to be a delightful little walled town with arched gateways, surrounded by acres of vineyards. There were narrow, cobbled streets and, in the centre, an open place. I found the hospital where the two doctors worked and also an untidy graveyard, but no indication of where the Daxs' had lived;

indeed there was nothing whatsoever to associate Dax *père* and Dax *fils* with Sommières.

A year or so later, I was invited to read a paper in Paris before the joint meeting of the Section of Neurology of the Royal Society of Medicine and the Societé Française de Neurologie. I chose the Dax-Broca controversy as my theme. I mentioned my visit to Sommières and my surprise at not finding any local recognition, even though many roads were endowed with eponyms. My remarks did not fall on stony ground.

Professor Passouant of Montpellier got in touch with the Mayor of Sommières, Monsieur André, himself a doctor. Contact was then made with Professor Alajouanine, who set about repairing the strange omission. On 12th June 1966, accompanied by Dr. Fergus Ferguson, whom Alajouanine had also invited, I travelled to Sommières. There was a reception at the Mairie, where Alajouanine said in his speech that the lack of recognition of their two honoured citizens constituted a kind of sclerosis, and, what was worse, he said, "*une sclerose sans plâques.*"

The meeting adjourned for a gargantuan luncheon, followed by more speeches. Next, we processed through the streets where flags were displayed at the windows, preceded by the band of the Fire Brigade. Inevitably, the scene was reminiscent of Chevalier's "Clochemerle".

The procession halted in a narrow street. Young ladies with bouquets stepped forward, and Alajouanine pulled a cord to reveal a plaque denoting the domicile of Dr. Marc Dax. That was not all. We snaked through more streets to the market place. There were more girls with bouquets, and I unveiled a plaque proclaiming that we were now in the Place Docteur Marc Dax et Docteur Gustave Dax, formerly Place du Marché.

Alajouanine was fond of entertaining, usually at his fine apartment on the first floor of the Avenue Victor Hugo. Here were displayed his many pictures; his study resembled a section of the London Library. Sometimes he took me out to lunch or dinner. Once he told me we would be having lunch the following day and asked whether I would like any special dish. Mindful of delicious meals in Cahors and in Toulouse, I requested cassoulet. Alajouanine's perpetual smile deepened. The next day we were lunching in a cosy restaurant near Les Halles. The beans, pork and goose went down well, and Alajouanine introduced me that day to Sancerre, a wine which I have never ceased to enjoy.

Afterwards he said he would take me to inspect a little Burgundian restaurant. It was situated in one of the smallest roads in old Paris. As we entered, the *patron* came forward. Alajouanine explained that we were not stopping; he wanted only to show me the picture. On the wall was a large colour-print in the style of Toulouse-Lautrec depicting a couple at the Bal Tabarin. The man was holding the girl under her armpits from behind, while she was executing the splits. Beneath was the legend—obviously a quotation—"A book opens easily at the most read page."

We continued to wander through the Latin Quarter until we found ourselves in the rue des Beaux Arts. Knowing my interest in Wildeana, Alajouanine took me to the Hotel d'Alsace, where Wilde had died. Awed no doubt by the red and white rosette in Alajouanine's buttonhole, denoting that he was a Grand Officier of the Légion d'Honneur, the proprietor was eager to oblige us. We saw the bedroom with adjoining small sitting-room looking out upon an attractive courtyard with a solitary tree. These were the rooms Wilde had referred to as "one for sleeping in and the other for my insomnia. More accurately, both are for my insomnia." Looking around, we could but remember the last words Wilde was alleged to have spoken: "This wallpaper is killing me: one or other of us must go."

On another occasion after lunch, he suggested that we should visit an art exhibition, which gave us the opportunity of gazing at an amazing collection of paintings by Modigliani.

Alajouanine always had an aura of calm. His voice was quiet and rather high-pitched. He was a taciturn person, and his students were accustomed to spells of reflective silence in his clinic. Unlike so many of his countrymen, he was not imbued with the desire to communicate with expansive gestures of limbs and trunk. His sole motor activity was his perpetual rolling of untidy cigarettes, his gaze fixed ahead of him and always silent.

His equanimity was superbly demonstrated when, in 1949, he chaired the important business meeting at the end of the 3rd International Congress of Neurology in Paris. The subject of debate was the location of the next Congress four years ahead. Rival offers were put forward in several different languages and a frenzy of gesticulation. Fists were shaken. Pandemonium broke out and violence seemed imminent. Some delegates slipped out to make telephone calls to their Embassies, and came back with extravagant promises. Throughout all this, Alajouanine stood, silent, with his perpetual pussy-cat smile, rolling a cigarette. Eventually, the hubbub subsided and he pronounced his final and decisive word—"Lisbon".

For me personally, Alajouanine did so much, and his generosity extended to my family. My son fell victim to an attack of poliomyelitis which was severe enough to prevent his doing National Service in the Army. He was, therefore, left with a year to spare before taking up his place at Oxford. Alajouanine arranged for him to enter the Sorbonne for the twelve-month course of Civilization Française. He was invited to spend some time at Alajouanine's country retreat, La Chalouze, in the heart of the department of Allier. Alajouanine lived in faded splendour in his book-filled country house, and demonstrated to Julian his unusual knowledge of edible fungi abounding in the nearby woods. It was to this house that he retired when he relinquished the Charcot Chair, passing his time reading and, sometimes, writing.

On his 80th birthday, a party was arranged in his honour at the Salpêtrière. I eagerly made the journey to Paris, only to learn that he was not well enough to attend. But a message awaited me to take tea with him in the Avenue Victor Hugo.

He was there with two or three other friends, and we drank his health in champagne.

Ten years later, the invitation was given in reverse on my 80th birthday for him to attend the celebrations in London. Alajouanine promised to come and to read a paper about his old and revered friend, Charles Foix. Alas, now 90, Alajouanine could not manage it. He died shortly afterwards, peacefully, in his beloved Chalouze, not far from where he was born.

I mourned the loss of my friend of half a century, but both of us had outlived the Biblical allotted span. Medical historians will deeply regret that his appreciation of Charles Foix never materialised. We have been deprived of a tribute to that brilliant poet-physician Charles Foix, from the pen of his closest friend and admirer, Théophile Alajouanine.

1905–1983
Morris B. Bender

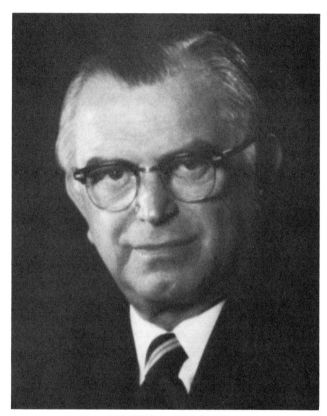

MORRIS B. BENDER

Courtesy of Mrs. Sara Bender.

Although I have often been accused of ancestor-worship (as though that were some unseemly heresy), I have also been able to recognise special abilities in my contemporaries. One person who stood out conspicuously among those who were younger than me was Morris Bender.

We did not meet until the Second World War had ended. Both of us had been Naval surgeons, but my peregrinations had not at that time taken me to San Diego, where he was stationed. I was drawn to his work at a time when I was involved in the symptomatology of parietal lesions. Independently, each of us had realised that simultaneous bilateral tactile stimulation often seemed to be perceived on one side only. To Morris Bender this was "tactile extinction", while I had used the expression "tactile inattention". Terminology was the sole point on which we did not agree.

My many post-war visits to America always took me to New York, where I never failed to make contact with Morris. Thus began a deep friendship, with considerable admiration on my part and great warmth and hospitality on his. I made many attempts to persuade him to visit London and to lecture, but he was a very busy man. However, as Dean of the Institute of Neurology, I eventually had the pleasure of presiding at a lecture given by him in London, and of introducing him to a large audience. In my opening remarks I told the students that Morris and I were friends, whose sole disagreement was one of nomenclature and reminded them of the rabbi who said to the cardinal, "Why should we quarrel? After all, we both serve the same God—you in your way and I in His."

Every time I was in New York, I attended his rounds at

Mount Sinai Hospital. Here I witnessed a feast, a performance such as one rarely sees nowadays. Morris's interrogation of a patient was gentle but deeply probing; some of his questions were unexpected. His thorough physical examination often included novel methods of approach, testifying to the originality of his thinking.

At that time, Bender often collaborated with the clinical psychologist Hans-Lukas Teuber, who had been a Pharmacist in the San Diego Naval Hospital during the war. Teuber was a pleasant, intelligent and enthusiastic colleague, and his association with Bender was a fruitful one. Teuber, alas, was to die prematurely in tragic circumstances.

But there was never a lack of able co-workers, for Bender's researches attracted the zeal of many young graduates who were later to achieve distinction in their own right.

As his writings show, Morris Bender made himself the supreme authority upon the intricacies of the oculomotor apparatus, an interest possibly instigated by his apprenticeship with Spiller and encouraged by Fulton.

Morris and his charming wife Sara were warmly hospitable to me. We either went together to a Broadway theatre or to their delightful house at Great Neck, Long Island, where Sara presided over delicious Russian-Jewish dinners. When the weather was propitious, the Benders held supper parties on the lawns which led down to the water. Many interesting guests were invited, and I remember meeting Jonathan Miller there on one occasion. I had known his father, Emmanuel Miller, the psychiatrist, and we had visited the Soviet Union together in 1931. Jonathan had interrupted his medical studies and was appearing on the stage in New York in "Beyond the Fringe".

The choice of venue was left to Morris. Once we attended the first night of *Camelot*, followed by a party at the St. Regis Hotel. Another time, Morris—or was it his secretary—booked seats at the Martin Beck Theatre. We sat grimly through *The Persecution and Assassination of Marat as Performed by the Inmates of the Asylum of Charenton Under the Direction of the Marquis de Sade.*

The title had intrigued us, but we felt cheated. The theme was too like "shop", and we considered we should have received a fat fee for our attendance.

Morris usually invited me to talk to his students, and it was on one of my visits that I was asked to deliver an Israel Wechsler lecture. Here I met many of Bender's former pupils like Edwin Weinstein, S.P. Diamond, Stefan Schanzer and many others; also some of his seniors, such as Wechsler and Goldstein. Once I was pleased to detect in the audience the former assistant of Schuster of Berlin, Dr. Pinéas.

Morris spoke little about his upbringing and early medical career. In time I learned that he was born in Uman, a small industrial town in the Ukraine, and that his parents took him to America when he was nine years of age. They settled in Philadelphia, where he attended school. Times were hard, and young Bender did several part-time jobs to help out. Later, when at University, he did night duty at the Post Office. At first he studied engineering, for he was good at mathematics. He quickly changed, however, to the Faculty of Medicine.

Among his teachers was the renowned W.G. Spiller, who had earlier spent four postgraduate years in Europe. Spiller had thus been a pupil of Gowers and also of Edinger and Oppenheim, and much of this experience must have been transmitted to the young Bender. Later, he studied neurophysiology with John Fulton at Yale, neuropathology with Globus, and psychiatry with that brilliant representative of the Vienna school, Paul Schilder.

Where did Morris Bender acquire his quite exceptional skill as a doctor in his search to unravel the nature of the obscure symptoms and physical signs presented by his anxious, bemused patients? Spiller no doubt played an important role, and, later still, Wechsler. But the fire in Morris's belly was mainly self-ignited.

Morris Bender was endowed with a deep interest in perceptual disorders. His important contributions to the field of both visual and tactile perception were highly original and exciting.

He employed novel methods of examination, and these, in turn, evoked surprising results. In my opinion, these papers constitute a great addition to the corpus of neurology. It was good to find that he shared my scepticism as to the notion of pure visual object agnosia. Furthermore, his experiences with that odd visual aberration—palinopsia—made most agreeable reading for me.

He was no blind follower of what was traditional. He did not hesitate at times to query observations and ideas that had been taken for granted. His thinking was refreshingly individualistic.

Morris had a large and loving family, and a hoard of loyal ex-students. He was much in demand as a consultant. Despite his popularity, he was free from pomposity, ostentation or conceit. There was something essentially boyish about him—a trait which he shared with two other great men I knew, Luria and Garcin.

One reason for his success was his caring attitude, to use an over-worked cliché. He exuded sympathy and understanding. He protected his patients from meddlesome invasive investigations, and especially from the intervention of eager neurosurgeons. For example, a subdural haematoma was not, in his opinion, a condition that called for instant surgery. Furthermore, Morris had a conservative attitude towards cerebral tumours. His patients with malignant growths in their brains were usually treated with radiotherapy and steroids rather than surgery. In his opinion, his patients' lives were thereby made more endurable.

On 8th May 1968, Morris Bender, Chairman of the Department of Neurology at the Mount Sinai School of Medicine, was appointed to the first Henry P. and Georgette Goldschmid Chair of Neurology. I was invited to New York to attend the investiture and to deliver the principal address. This was a memorable occasion.

When the ceremony was over, the principal guests were taken to a hotel. A dining table was laid for us in a smallish room and Morris and I, and a handful of others, drank our martinis.

When the time came to sit down at the table, we found our place-cards and awaited the first course. Suddenly, a screen which covered the whole of one wall was thrown back, to reveal a large dining room filled with round tables at which were seated at least a hundred of his former students, past interns, assistants and friends. The disclosure was dramatic, for none of us at Morris's table had any inkling that the hospitality was to be on such a scale.

In 1972 Morris Bender presided over the annual meeting of the American Neurological Association in Chicago. His Presidential address was an unusual one, though topical. His subject was "Perceptual Interaction and Acupuncture Anaesthesia".

The last time I saw Morris at work, he demonstrated to me with great clarity the value of graphaesthesia in the diagnosis of parietal disease. Hitherto I had been sceptical about the alleged value of this test, the components of which entail so many variables. In Morris's hands, however, there was a consistency in his method of carrying out the manoeuvre that was impressive. I became convinced that graphaesthesia could be a useful adjunct to one's battery of tests for perceptual disorders.

On 24th January 1983, I was seeing patients in my consulting rooms in London, when Morris's secretary telephoned me from New York to tell me that he had died suddenly the previous day. She said she knew Morris would not have liked me to learn about his death fortuitously. As he would have chosen, he was working hard when he died, and he was spared the affliction of ill-health and also the tedium of eroding senescence.

During my neurological career I have been fortunate in knowing many clinicians of distinction. Morris Bender stands firmly among the greatest of them. He possessed the qualities which Nathaniel Hawthorne rated so highly in a physician— native sagacity, intuition and lack of intrusive egotism. He was endowed with the power that was surely born in him, of bringing his mind into affinity with his patients.

1872–1934
Gaétan Gatian de Clérambault

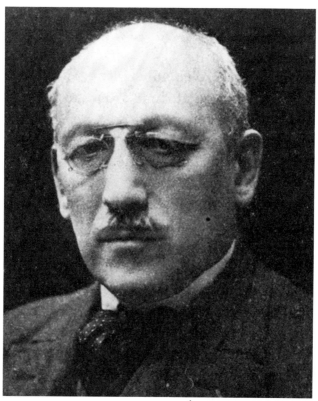

GAÉTAN GATIAN DE **CLÉRAMBAULT**

Courtesy of the National Library of Medicine, Washington, D.C.

This aristocratic name—evocative of the age of elegance—may be familiar today to some informed psychiatrists, but probably not to many neurologists even in France. He occupies an important niche in my memory, for it was he who was responsible for my first visit to Paris. The year was 1928. To him I owe the beginnings of my lifelong admiration for French neurology.

My visit came about in an unusual manner. As a Medical Registrar, I had published an unpretentious monograph upon the enigmatic subject of mirror-writing (*Mirror-Writing*. London: Kegan Paul, Trubner, Trench & Co., 1928). This paramedical curiosity led to my meeting three unusual individuals—J.D. Rolleston, F.G. Crookshank and C.K. Ogden.

The first of these erudite men was the brother of the President of the Royal College of Physicians, Regius Professor of Physic at Cambridge, and Physician to the King. J.D. was a quiet, retiring, studious man, whose post as Superintendent of a fever hospital gave him abundant time for literary and historical research. Among his unorthodox writings were a medical commentary upon the works of Rabelais, and a startling dissertation on Penis Captivus.

Dr. Crookshank was a psychiatrist interested in migraine. His was the aphorism that a migrainous attack represents the product of baffled rage and humiliation. His classic *The Mongol in Our Midst* brought him fame.

C.K. Ogden was an eccentric psycholinguistic philosopher. He was the co-author of the important monograph *The Meaning of Meaning*. But he is probably best remembered as the inventor of Basic English—an attempt at a universal language founded upon 850 simple English key words.

As a result of my contact with these learned pedagogues, it was suggested that I should visit Paris and lecture (in English) upon the subject of mirror-writing. My host would be Clérambault, at whose clinic I would give a talk. A date in March 1928 was decided upon.

Clérambault's clinic was held each morning in the Infirmerie Speciale within the Palais de Justice on the Ile de la Cité. Here were housed a police headquarters and a remand prison. The police referred to the clinic some of the individuals, picked up the day before, whose behaviour had been not only anti-social but slightly crazy. It was Clérambault's task to identify those offenders who presented genuine psychiatric problems. The clinic was officially recognised as a venue for postgraduate students and would-be psychiatrists. It was extremely popular, for Clérambault was a dramatic diagnostician and an exciting and original teacher.

There one might meet such characters as those who expose themselves *coram publico;* some shoplifters and pick-pockets; hooligans indulging in noisy conduct in the streets; those found unconscious in the gutter, perhaps in convulsions; would-be suicides; youngsters more than usually high on marihuana; the drunks who were far too disorderly; and persons accused of unwarranted aggression.

Such a morning parade of flashers, dippers, brawlers, fitters, streakers and junkies would be interviewed, adjourned for further information, arraigned, hospitalised, or even recommended for release. Dr. de Clérambault was all-powerful.

I accepted the invitation with alacrity and wrote to Clérambault giving the title and summary of my paper, informing him, too, that I had many illustrations to project. The idea of extending my time in Paris and combining an exploration of the city with a visit to a number of hospitals and neurologists occurred to me. It was a particularly favourable time to visit France, for the rate of exchange was very much in our favour.

I was put up at the modest Hôtel Corneille, in the Latin Quarter near the Odéon. No one met me at the railway station.

I showed up at the Palais de Justice just before the appointed hour. Clérambault greeted me heartily and conducted me to the lecture theatre, where already some early visitors were seated. I handed my host my pile of 30 or so glass lantern slides arranged in appropriate order. He said, "What are they for? We haven't got a projector of any sort, and it is too late to borrow one." This was a blow, because I doubted whether many in the audience understood English, and I was relying heavily on visual aids.

My lecture comprised a succession of simple sentences, slowly and deliberately articulated. After a paragraph or two I paused and handed my first 5 cm by 5 cm lantern slide to the person seated at one end of the front row. The recipient would hold the slide up to the light, peer at it intently and then pass it on to his neighbour. Then came a few more sentences and another slide. Slowly the illustrations went the rounds of the audience, but the gap between the spoken word and its illustration became longer and longer.

I was invited by Clérambault to lunch with him the next day. He lived on the periphery of Paris in Malakoff, an area which was then more rural than urban. I was given detailed instructions how to get to his house. I found a half built-up road, flanked by a high wall, and then I came upon a door in the wall and a bell-pull. I tugged at the handle and heard it clanging in the distance. A long interval followed. Should I try again? It reminded me of visits I paid to convents to see sick nuns, especially when I heard footsteps approaching. The door was opened by a beautiful girl of about 18. "You wish to see Dr. de Clérambault? Come inside." I advanced along lengthy garden paths and then corridors, until I found myself within a veritable Arabian tent. The girl left me there and I did not see her again. I saw prayer-mats on the floor; carpets hanging from the walls; scimitars and shields; texts from the Koran. On the tables were prayer-beads and other artefacts. All around were Muslim trappings. My host appeared and conducted me to the dinner table.

The cuisine was excellent and wine flowed freely. As the conversation progressed, Clérambault's diction became faster and faster, and it was increasingly difficult for me to interpret the gist of his conversation. Presumably it was political and dealt with Anglo-French post-war relationships. My grounds for this belief was the frequent occurrence of the words "Lloyd George". Much else was over my head.

My host eventually tired of his monologue, and he diverted my attention to what was obviously his principal interest, namely the philosophy of clothing throughout the ages. He took me around his house, where there stood "dummies" such as one sees in shop windows. They were dressed in a variety of costumes; here an ancient Greek chiton; an Indian sari or dhoti; a Roman toga; there a Moroccan dishdash, as well as medieval costumes. Apparently, Clérambault was engaged in writing a magnum opus on the subject of *La Draperie*, which he hoped would constitute the definitive work upon the subject.

Clérambault went on to comment upon the asymmetry of the method of putting on clothes in various regions of the world. Why does a woman fasten her coat with the buttons on the left, while a man buttons his clothes from right to left? In the case of the Indian sari, a rectangular piece of cotton or silk, 5 to 7 yards in length, would be held at the left-hand extremity, laid against the front of the body and held tightly in place, while the remainder was wrapped around the body in an anti-clockwise direction, finishing with the end over the left shoulder or perhaps the head. Presumably, said Clérambault, this asymmetry was a result of inequality of function of the two cerebral hemispheres and reflected the common left-brain dominance. He claimed he had met some women who wore their saris the wrong way round—presumably they were left-handed, although he was not sure.

His cogitating proceeded to a consideration of the Scottish kilt, which is also wrapped anti-clockwise around the pelvis. Could it be that somewhere in Scotland there might be a left-handed Highlander whose kilt was worn mirror-fashion, he mused.

The party broke up late; I was due to meet the Dean of the Faculty, Gustave Roussy. I did not expect to see Clérambault again. None of my neurological contacts in Paris was able to tell me much about this eccentric but kindly character. Psychiatric friends in England told me a little more.

Gaétan Gatian de Clérambault was born in the heart of France in the historic town of Bourges. Originally he had been destined for a legal career, but he qualified in medicine. He then specialised in psychiatry, and more especially in the forensic aspects of his discipline. In 1905 he became assistant to Dupré at the Infirmerie Spéciale des Aliénés du Préfecture de Police at the Palais de Justice, becoming Médecin-Chef in 1921.

From what I subsequently learned, Clérambault had contributed to the corpus of psychiatry some interesting and novel ideas. His early studies were on patients addicted to such drugs as chloral, ether and hashish. Next came his conception of mental automatism, whereby certain mental states could exist in detachment. Another phenomenon associated with his name is the notion of *psychoses passionelles*. A powerful emotion, anger perhaps, or lust, or jealousy, or a sense of grievance, may lead to a delusional state. This ideo-affective linkage becomes established. No hallucinations arise and there is no thought-disorder.

At a time when it seemed as though psychiatry might be submerged by psychological, philosophical and psychoanalytical theories, Clérambault became the head of a group of dissidents who regarded psychiatry as an expansion of general medicine.

Apparently there has recently been something of a revival of interest in Clérambault's conjectures, both in France and in Great Britain.

Two years later I met Clérambault again in Paris. After that, the lectures, meetings and dinners that I attended in France were mainly neurological and Clérambault was not present. From time to time I enquired of my friends about him. They seemed to regard him as a clever man, an original thinker, but unconventional. The last I heard of him was in 1934, when I was told that he had committed suicide. As far as I could determine, his projected tome on the philosophy of clothing was never completed.

Many years later I learned more about this intriguing man. He was a member of an illustrious family, which included such notables as a cardinal of the Church of Rome, a Marshal of the French Army, the philosopher René Descartes, the poet Alfred de Vigny and at least one member of the Académie Française. Dr. de Clérambault was universally regarded as a man of exceptionally high intelligence. One admirer stated that he had an insight into the mind of the insane that was uncanny. He was a solitary individual and a bachelor, and he was regarded as being aloof and abrasive except with a few close friends. To these he sometimes spoke of himself as "that old paranoiac".

During the first World War he served with considerable bravery in a battalion of Moroccan sharpshooters and was twice wounded. In order to form a sympathetic bond with his troops, he learned Arabic. Many times after the war he visited Morocco.

Clérambault's contributions to psychiatry were highly original and essentially organismic. He was largely out of sympathy with contemporary trends in thinking. He was anxious to communicate his viewpoint in detail to a wider audience, but unfortunately failing eyesight made his task increasingly difficult. An operation for bilateral cataract proved unsuccessful. During his convalescence he became bedridden from arthritis. Obviously he would never witness the culmination of his life's work. He decided to terminate what he regarded as his useless existence.

A conspicuous figure at his funeral was General Pellerin, who had been his commanding officer and who wished to pay respects to the passing of his outstandingly courageous colleague.

Eight years after his death, a number of his ex-pupils and friends published Clérambault's works under the title *Oeuvre Psychiatrique* edited by Jean Fretit and issued by the Presses

Universitaires de Paris. A thoughtful preface was contributed by Dr. Paul Guiraud.

What solace it would have been to Clérambault in his latter days of sightless and painful loneliness had he been made aware of the loyal action of his former pupils. Perhaps, too, he would have chuckled had he also known that fifty years later young psychiatrists are writing theses upon his very personal contributions to the study of mental disorders.

In an obituary Dr. Henyer quoted some verses written by Clérambault's kinsman, Comte Alfred de Vigny, and I can find nothing more fitting as my own tribute:

J'ai mis sur le cimier doré du gentilhomme
Une plume de fer qui n'est pas sans beauté.
J'ai fait illustre un nom qu'on m'a transmis sans gloire.
Qu'il soit ancien qu'importe? Il n'aura de memoire
Que du jour seulement ou mon front l'a porté.

(Upon my gold crest of nobility
I had placed a plume of iron of no little beauty.
I have brought lustre to a name inherited in its simplicity.
What matter that it be of ancient lineage? It will be remembered
Only because of the strength I have brought to it.)

1922–1986
Irving S. Cooper

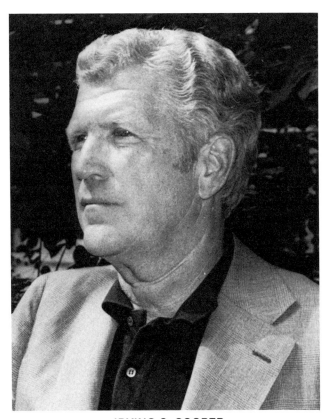

IRVING S. COOPER

Courtesy of Mrs. Sissel Cooper.

We first met on 22nd July 1957, during the VIth International Congress of Neurology in Brussels. Professor van Gehuchten, the President, invited me to a small dinner party at his home, and Irving Cooper was also among the guests. I had heard of him as a surgeon who had been successful in treating patients disabled by Parkinson's disease by means of a stereotactic approach. Such operations were not then widely carried out in England, and I had no experience as to its efficacy.

Irving Cooper was a most agreeable table-companion. It transpired that each of us had served as Naval officers during the war—something which never fails to establish an empathy. The conversation at dinner was about this and that, the topic of neurology scarcely arising. Somehow the name of Dylan Thomas, who had recently died in New York, arose. We talked about his work *Under Milk Wood*. It had been recorded in America, and I said it was not yet available in England. Immediately he promised to send the records to me when he returned home. I thought no more about it until a few weeks later when, to my surprise and delight, a set of records arrived with a gracious letter inviting me to visit his clinic next time I was in New York. In the meantime, I had learned a little more of what Cooper was doing.

Neurologists had long been aware that, should a patient with Parkinson's disease happen to sustain a stroke, the tremor in the paralysed limbs would be eradicated. In the recent past, attempts had been made to abolish extrapyramidal rigidity and tremor by ablation of the voluntary motor pathways at various levels in the neuraxis. Experience had shown that these two symptoms could not be overcome save by the imposition of paralysis. Cooper, always a pioneer refusing to be shackled by convention, thought that an assault upon the motor pathways might be worth trying if carried out at an unusual site, namely where they entered the internal capsule. His patient was a man severely crippled by a post-encephalitic syndrome. At that date, October 1951, Cooper had no personal surgical service but he had access to facilities in Bellevue Hospital, New York.

The operation began. The dura was opened and the cerebral hemisphere retracted to permit access to the basal regions. At this point, troublesome bleeding occurred and it became necessary to clamp the anterior choroidal artery. Cooper decided to proceed no further with the operation. On the patient recovering from the anaesthetic, it was found to everyone's astonishment that the tremor in the opposite arm and leg was no longer present. The rigidity too had been replaced by flaccidity and, wonder of wonders, the patient was able to move the limb and even carry out coordinated movements.

Was this the result of a cutting-off of the blood supply to that small, deep-seated area supplied by the anterior choroidal artery? Would the same benefit accrue if this measure were carried out in other patients?

Here, indeed, was a case of serendipity. But, as Pasteur observed long ago, discoveries are made by a mind that is prepared. Otherwise the whole event might pass unnoticed. Professor Austen of Denver prefers to use the term he coined, "altamirage", rather than serendipity. It derives from the experience of archeologists in Northern Spain, whose knowledge of the local geology led them to believe that somewhere close by must be a considerable cavernous formation. One day a terrier chased a rabbit to its bolt-hole. The archeologists followed, opened up the gap in the rocky surface, and stumbled upon the now world-famous cave of Altamira.

From my own earlier work upon the blood-supply of the brain, I knew that, phylogenetically speaking, the anterior choroidal artery was one of the oldest and most interesting blood vessels in the mammalian brain. It represents the posterior branch of the cranial carotid and, consequently, in the more lowly vertebrates constitutes the principal supply of blood to the primitive brain.

Irving Cooper was tempted to repeat this operation. A likely candidate was found in a severely affected post-encephalitic patient, who was in an institution for those afflicted with chronic disorders. The Medical Superintendent was reluctant to permit such an experimental venture, but the patient's relatives were strongly in favour of the idea. Five months after Cooper's original operation, this patient submitted to surgery. The anterior choroidal artery was found to be too tenuous for silver clips to be applied, and was, therefore, coagulated by diathermy.

Again, an excellent clinical result followed.

Over the ensuing months, eleven similar patients were treated. Six of them markedly improved; one died. Four patients were not materially helped.

Irving Cooper reported his findings at the annual meeting of The American Neurological Association in June, 1953. He received a mixed reception from the physicians present. Considerable attention was aroused in the lay Press, especially *The New York Times*. A Pandora's box had been opened letting out a number of Trojan horses, as Ernest Bevin, the British Foreign Secretary, is reputed to have said in quite another connection.

Overnight Irving Cooper became a well-known but controversial figure. Hundreds of patients were referred to him, and his post-operative results were, in most cases, strikingly favourable. Three consequences followed: persistent attention from the Press; disapproval by many of his colleagues; and the acquisition of wealth. Not all neurologists and neurosurgeons were antagonistic, and many of the medical profession in America and abroad were strongly supportive.

These events were unknown to me when I first met Cooper, but I came to realise that among my close friends in the U.S.A. were some who were hostile to him. They did not openly say so to me, and his name was rarely, if ever, mentioned in my presence.

Cooper later decided to abandon ligation of the choroidal artery and substitute a simple stereotactic necrotisation of the presumed area of significance.

The first chemopallidectomy was carried out in December 1953 in the presence of a distinguished visitor, Sir Geoffrey Jefferson. "Cooper", he said, "there is no question in my mind that the results are valid and important". He went on to warn Cooper, however, that he would probably encounter no little scepticism.

By this time Cooper sorely needed facilities for his surgical work, and eventually found in the Bronx an old, unattractive "Home for Incurables" that had been built at a time when that area was farmland. The Board of Governors offered him accommodation in that hospital, and alterations were made to provide for him an office, a tiny operating room and two six-bedded wards. The institution's name was changed and it became St. Barnabas' Hospital.

The next juncture in the stereotactic saga was the realisation that the factor that brought relief to the symptoms of Parkinsonism was a lesion not in the globus pallidas but in the ventrolateral region of the thalamus. The operation of choice now became a chemothalamectomy.

Cooper later devised a method of necrotising part of the thalamus by freezing the tissue with liquid nitrogen. Apparently there were many technical advantages in this operation of cryothalamectomy. The first patient to be so treated was in 1961 or 1962; the precise date is not clear.

It was at this stage that I first visited St. Barnabas' Hospital. Cooper sent his car and driver to my hotel in Manhattan, and I was taken through a rather run-down area of the Bronx to the hospital. Cooper greeted me in the entrance hall. He was a tall, handsome, athletic man with crisp, close-cut blond hair. We went to his office, which was crowded with books, papers, X-ray viewing boxes and a closed-circuit television screen connected with the operating theatre. In the course of a highly interesting talk, he explained his technique for the relief of tremor and rigidity in Parkinsonians. He did not claim that the natural progression of the disease was halted, but the extent of palliation that followed was dramatic.

By 1961, three thousand patients had been operated upon, the vast majority being considerably improved. The immediate mortality was low. Some cases were complicated by a cerebro-vascular insult some days or weeks later.

Cooper contemplated employing cryosurgery in an attempt to cure other movement-disorders, such as severe intention tremor, senile tremor, athetosis and torticollis. Furthermore, by repeated cryosurgical interferences, he was tackling cases of torsion dystonia.

Each patient in his clinic was examined and recorded in considerable detail, and cinematography was used routinely. Around him, Cooper had assembled a team of assistants and advisers, including interns, medical neurologists, speech therapists, psychologists and psychiatrists. In his work he was collaborating with Dr. Robert Schwab of Boston and Professor Rusk, Chief of the New York Rehabilitation Service.

Cooper invited me to watch him carry out a cryothalamectomy upon a patient with Parkinson's disease. The patient was conscious throughout, but at no time showed any sign of pain or discomfort. The insulated probe was inserted a distance of about 2½ inches, X-ray pictures being repeatedly taken to demonstrate the orientation of the instrument. When the target was reached, a limited degree of freezing was carried out. The patient's upper limb was closely observed. His tremor ceased and the fingers relaxed, so that the spasm of the hand was overcome. Cooper told the patient to move his fingers, then his wrist and arm. It was obvious that the probe was in position; a little more liquid nitrogen was introduced and the probe then removed. The whole procedure was carried out quietly, quickly, smoothly and with a *coup de maître* that was astonishing.

By 1968, that is over a period of 15 years, Cooper and his team had operated upon more than eight thousand patients.

My first visit was followed by many meetings during the next 25 years. Apart from being a skilful surgeon, I discovered Cooper to be a remarkable man of many abilities; in fact, he was quite exceptional. Towards me he was hospitable, generous and warm-hearted. I stayed in his lovely house in Pelham Manor, Westchester, outside New York City, where he enjoyed having lavish parties. He took me out in his 42-foot craft "The Matador". For years he had used this means of commuting between Pelham Manor and Bellevue Hospital.

Irving Cooper, I learned, was born in Atlantic City, New Jersey, on 15th July 1922. He did well at school, entered college at Syracuse, and then studied at George Washington University. There he met Dr. Walter Freeman, whose dynamism directed Cooper's interest towards neurology. In Cooper's own words: "I literally fell in love with the brain: its structure, its functions (at that time largely unknown), its complexity and the miraculous creation that it is." Part of his medical apprenticeship was spent in the U.S. Navy, and he learned his neurosurgery at the Mayo Clinic.

Outside neurology, Cooper and I had at least one interest in common, namely a preoccupation with language and languages. I subsequently learned from him that as a schoolboy he was much influenced by a teacher who aroused in him an interest in words. How fortunate he was, for teachers of that type are rare, but their powers of moulding the minds and careers of those youngsters who are receptive, are enormous. At George Washington University he fell under the spell of Professor Fred Tupper of the English Department. As Cooper was later to write: "Fred Tupper was a great teacher. He did not just teach the plays of Shakespeare, he interpreted the temper of his time, the meaning of his language, the rhythm and poetry of his thought . . . I can close my eyes and see Fred Tupper, book in hand, but without any need to refer to it, acting out in front of our class, teaching us what lay behind each line, describing the spontaneous overflow of powerful feelings poetically expressed by Shakespeare, teaching us the origins of the history and emotions of the characters, giving us a gift that would last an entire lifetime ... Professor Tupper was a profound and great teacher. No classroom teacher has had a greater or more lasting influence upon my life."

Cooper's interest in language was not confined to the English tongue. At one time he became fascinated with all things pertaining to Spain—the country, its history, culture, food, wine and, in particular, the literature. He employed Spanish-speaking teachers and secretaries, and he selected some of his surgical assistants from Latin America. Later on, he surrounded himself with Italian-speaking staff; still later, it was the Russian language that preoccupied him.

Some of Cooper's brief leisure time was occupied in writing. He made many contributions to surgical and medical journals. In addition, he published books entitled, *The Victim is Always the Same, Living with Chronic Neurological Disease,* and a novel dealing with a medico-ethical theme which he called *It's Hard to Leave While the Music's Playing.* In 1980, he sent to me in London the typescript of his projected autobiography. I was fascinated but shocked by parts of it. He had written with considerable bitterness about several distinguished medical men whom I admired and who were also friends of mine. I thought that, in places, the terminology he had used was quite unacceptable.

I advised Cooper not to publish the book. After some weeks, I had a letter saying he had decided to go ahead with its publication, but he had drastically toned down the episodes to which I had referred. In 1981, *The Vital Probe* appeared, published by Norton and Company.

We were both interested in paintings. I had met Peter Curtis, the surrealist artist of Scottsdale, Arizona, and had bought one of his works. Cooper and I spent a pleasant afternoon visiting an exhibition of Curtis's paintings in New York, and going into one art gallery after another along Madison Avenue. Regrettably, he did not buy a Curtis.

In June 1975, Cooper invited me to stay in his delightful new house at Onteora, in a lovely, wooded area in the Catskill Mountains in New York State. My wife and I spent some time there with him and his beautiful Norwegian second wife, Sissel. One memorable day, Coop—as he liked to be called—my wife and I set off to explore the numerous antique shops in nearby Connecticut. Coop bought a spinning wheel for Sissel, and we picked up some pieces of Staffordshire ware decorated with the name of my home town in England. It was a wonderful carefree time.

Coop often came to England, once staying in London for a six months' sabbatical. We met frequently then at the National Hospital and at dinner-parties. He had many loyal friends in Great Britain, including Sir Peter Medawar, the eminent bioscientist. We had close mutual friends in C.P. Snow, the philosopher-writer, and his wife, Pamela Hansford Johnson (Lord and Lady Snow).

In 1974, my wife and I wanted to make a token recognition of his kindness and friendship. We decided to give him "Yorick". Some time before, I had acquired in Vienna one of the actual skulls collected by F.J. Gall at the turn of the 18th century. Gall had delineated and indicated on its surface the various cerebral "organs". I kept it in my consulting rooms in Queen Square, to the delight of small boys who saw it. Eileen and I presented it to Coop and said we hoped he would fare well at the Customs when he returned to New York. The British Customs Officers had been quite puzzled by it when I brought it into England. Coop was delighted, and he had it mounted and encased and kept it on his desk. After his death, Sissel kindly returned the skull to me, and Yorick is now before me as I write.

Irving Cooper was an empiricist, an innovator and a pragmatist. He referred to himself as an experimental brain surgeon. Though his work was physiologically and anatomically orientated, he could not be ranked as a scientist *sensu stricto*. At a meeting in London in June 1979, Professor Patrick Wall, part-author of the "gate theory" of pain, demanded to be told what was the basic justification for making the lesions in the patient Cooper had been describing.

Cooper replied: "I am somewhat puzzled by your request for a justification for alleviating the total incapacity of Mrs. M. . . . I am a doctor. It is my legal and moral responsibility to try to make sick people well . . . I have for many years refused to apologise for the therapeutic benefit of these operations simply because the results could not be immediately explained by laboratory or clinical scientists on the basis of existing physiologic ideas—ideas which ultimately were demonstrably false. If I may quote a remark that Sir Peter Medawar made to me earlier in this meeting, 'It is a doctor's job to do good. It is a scientist's job to explain the facts' . . . I invite Professor Wall, as a scientist, to examine the unprecedented facts emerging from this experiment to explain them. If the facts do not fit his present concepts, then he will have to rethink the concepts, because the facts will not change . . . these are the facts. If we cannot entirely explain them now, they will, nevertheless, not go away. Eventually we will understand them and they will teach us more about the brain. In the meantime they have made some sick people well—and that is the role of a doctor."

I had myself seen and examined Mrs. M. when she first attended Cooper's clinic in November 1970. She had had a carditis and a valve replacement, followed by a cerebral embolus that had lodged in the right side of her midbrain producing clinical features of both a Weber's and a Benedikt's syndrome. Irving Cooper performed a series of surgical attacks. First the dentate nucleus of the cerebellum was destroyed, followed in two weeks by a cryothalamectomy. Six months later a right-sided pulvinarectomy was carried out. Two weeks after the third operation Mrs. M. walked out of the hospital to resume her normal life as a housewife.

A year after the first operation, however, the patient developed fatal bacterial endocarditis. Her brain was sent to the National Hospital for detailed study. A small lesion was found in the right half of the midbrain involving the reticular substance, the red nucleus and the oculomotor nucleus. The pathologist, Dr. Marion Smith, could find no lesion of the pyramidal tract despite the presence during life of a Babinski sign.

In 1967 Coop was awarded the Galen Gold Medal for Therapeutics by the Society of Apothecaries of London. The occasion was a special one, for the Society was celebrating the 350th anniversary of its foundation by King James I. Two medals were awarded that year, the other recipient being Sir Peter Medawar. A gathering of distinguished colleagues continued the celebrations later that night at the Savoy Hotel. The following evening, a banquet was held at the Apothecaries Hall in the presence of Her Majesty, The Queen Mother, and the then Prime Minister, Mr. Harold Macmillan. Coop came as my guest. The evening finished late because the Queen Mother was in no hurry to leave. Afterwards, my neurosurgical colleague from the National Hospital, Harvey Jackson, offered to drive us the comparatively short distance to the Savoy Hotel, where Coop was staying. Unfortunately, soon after we started, the Rolls Royce refused to go any further. Eventually, Coop and I, still in white tie and tails and aided by an amused taxi driver, pushed the vehicle along the Embankment.

With the introduction of the drug L-Dopa, Cooper virtually abandoned his operation of cryothalamectomy in cases of Parkinson's disease. His acceptance of the superior merits of L-Dopa was immediate and unqualified. In 1968 he laid down that no surgical procedures would be carried out in his service on any patient with the disease for at least a year. The 700 patients on his waiting list were so informed, and they were told about the new medical developments.

Cooper became a close friend of the innovator of L-Dopa, Dr. George Cotzias. He continued to treat by stereotactic methods cases of localised or generalised dystonia. In his own words: "I have fought like hell to prove my point, but once I approached the summit I have turned away to look elsewhere for a new challenge." He now directed his attention to the cerebellum, an organ which he stimulated electrically. I saw nothing of this side of his work.

By about 1976 he had left St. Barnabas' Hospital. We never discussed the reason for his leaving, but it obviously was a painful experience for him. My own last visit to that hospital was in 1975, when Coop organised a lecture there in my honour. I was especially pleased that several of the leading neurologists in New York attended, despite their coolness to Coop personally. The lecture, entitled "The Role of Silence in Theater and Films", was given by Walter Kerr, the celebrated author and drama critic.

Cooper set up an experimental surgical service in a hospital in Westchester. Later, he established the Institute for Advanced Studies in Medicine and the Humanities in Naples, Florida. Coop gave up his house in Pelham Manor and moved to Naples, continuing to spend holidays at Onteora. We met and dined together with our wives whenever we were in New York or they were in London.

Our last meeting was in the fall of 1983. I had completed a lecturing assignment in North Carolina but had not been able to fit in a visit to Florida. Eileen and I were returning home in the QE2, and Coop flew to New York to meet us and to give us dinner at the Four Seasons. We were mourning the recent loss of our friends, Lord and Lady Snow.

We continued to correspond. He was interested in patients with gross involuntary movements or with dystonia, as well as electrical stimulation of the cerebellum in cases of intractable epilepsy. He had sustained some visual problems as the result of an accident, but he made light of his troubles.

Unexpectedly in 1986, I heard from Sissel that Coop had died on 13th October from a carcinoma of the lung.

Coop was an innovator who brought substantial symptomatic relief to many thousands of unhappy victims of a sinister and progressive malady, for which at that time no treatment was known.

Professor Adrian Upton, one of the last of his collaborators, wrote that Irving Cooper was "a brilliant and vulnerable man who lived a full and exciting life as one of the great pioneers of neurosurgery of this century. He will be remembered by all who knew him well, and time will allow a full and fair appreciation of his great contributions to neurosurgery and to patients suffering from chronic illness."

1901–1980
Derek Denny-Brown

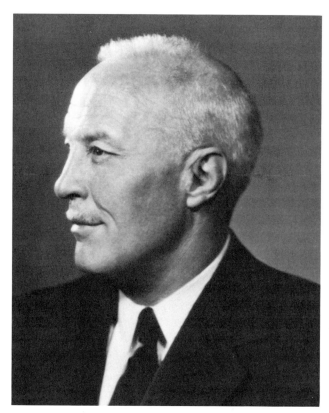

DEREK DENNY-BROWN

Courtesy of the Royal College of Physicians, London.

D enny-Brown came to the National Hospital as a House Physician in 1928, soon after I was appointed to the staff as Assistant Physician. It was obvious that his interests extended beyond clinical work into the application of physiology rather than bedside neurology, thus following the road taken by George Riddoch and F.M.R. Walshe. He worked hard, often late into the night, and the resources of Dr. Greenfield's pathological laboratory were available to him. He was essentially a do-it-yourself doctor, and worked up the morbid anatomy and histology of patients he had looked after. He hardened, cut, stained and mounted the specimens he needed and then carried out his own microphotography. It was not that he could not accept skilled assistance in these tasks, but he was compulsively self-sufficient. In this respect he resembled Kinnier Wilson, who went even further.

Denny-Brown was born in New Zealand, "that super suburbia of the Southern seas", as it has been rudely called, and came to Magdalen College, Oxford to learn his neurophysiology, having won a Beit Memorial Fellowship in 1925. The next three years were probably the most significant in his life. He became a pupil of Sherrington, the greatest figure in neurophysiology, and worked alongside Liddell and Creed, future Professors of Physiology, and Granit, who was to become a Nobel prize-winner.

He could have continued an academic career, and no doubt would have become a Fellow of the Royal Society or have even become a Nobel laureate. He could well have achieved a peerage, like Adrian. Instead, he elected to enter clinical neurology. I do not know whether someone dissuaded him from pursuing a scientific career, but his decision proved to be an advantage to neurology. Practising neurologists with a firm physiological foundation are rare indeed.

I found him to be a serious, dedicated individual with exceptional ability and drive, but he was also full of fun when off duty. He was in residence with other able young men who were more conventional. He persuaded one of them—Graeme Robertson—to collaborate with him on a study of bladder-function.

He did not then appear to be a dedicated clinician, if one bears in mind Moxon's dictates . . . "You must know diseases, not as a zoologist knows his species and his genera and his orders, by description of comparative characters, but as a hunter knows his lions and tigers." But Denny-Brown was no hunter, unlike Gowers, Holmes, Wilson, Adie, Symonds, Bender and Garcin. He was, as Dickens said, "a man of science, which is mother of invention, and knows no law". His dynamism was not the kind that led to the bedsides of tormented patients with neuropsychiatric disorders. He was a dissector.

His outstanding knowledge and abilities were recognised, and in due course he was appointed Assistant Physician to the National Hospital and also to St. Bartholomew's Hospital.

I have a vivid memory of Denny's residency at Queen Square. It was in 1931 that I first encountered a case of what came to be known as musicogenic epilepsy. My patient was a ward-maid at the hospital, and I had been treating her epilepsy for some years. Once when she attended Out-Patients, she mentioned to me, as an afterthought, that she only had an epileptic attack when she was listening to music. On pursuing the matter, I found that she was not musically enlightened; she said that not all kinds of music caused her to have a fit, but it was "classical" music that was dangerous.

She agreed to let me put her to the test, and she was admitted to the ward. I then had to provide the music. It transpired that Denny-Brown was the only person in Queen Square who owned a gramophone, so I borrowed it and his records. The first one

I played was a piece of jazz, but the patient said "It's not that sort that sets me off". I looked through the others, which were all of a similar type except one—Tchaikovsky's "Valse des Fleurs". After a few bars had been played, the patient had a grand mal seizure, during which both plantar responses changed from flexor to extensor. So, two points were established. First, musicogenic epilepsy did indeed exist. Secondly, Denny-Brown was then not a musical sophisticate.

I had a pleural effusion in 1933, and was off work for a time. Denny-Brown kindly agreed to be my *locum tenens* at a London County Council hospital, where I was the visiting neurologist. On one of his Saturday afternoon visits, the medical officer showed Denny a patient with extreme fatiguability, double vision and droopy eyelids, which he immediately recognised as a case of myasthenia gravis. The medical officer enquired as to the nature of this malady. Denny gave a succinct account of the characteristic signs and symptoms. "But what is the cause?", asked the M.O. The reply was to the effect that no one knew, nor was there any known treatment. "The picture", said Denny-Brown, "is rather like that of curare poisoning." After he had left the hospital, he told me, the medical officer consulted the toxicological section of her Burroughs Wellcome diary.

Returning to the ward, she prescribed physostigmine for the patient, who responded rapidly and temporarily improved. This was the beginning of our understanding and treatment of myasthenia.

Both of us were members of a small dining club, called The Hexagon. The other members were C.P. Symonds, George Riddoch, Hugh Cairns and Russell Brain. As I described in *The Citadel of the Senses* (Raven Press, 1985), we met to dine and afterwards one of us read a paper which was discussed critically by the others. Among the subjects contributed by Denny-Brown were cerebellar symptomatology; infective polyneuritis; lightning pains in neurosyphilitic patients other than tabetics; incoordinate ocular movements; and olivo-ponto-cerebellar atrophy.

In 1936 he went to Yale on a Rockefeller scholarship to work with John Fulton. He met many influential academics, who were greatly impressed by his scholarship and operosity, and by his deep knowledge of neurophysiology. On the retirement of Tracy Putnam in 1939, Denny-Brown was offered and took an appointment at Harvard.

The war broke out in September that year, and for the next six years I was in the Royal Navy, but we met once early in 1945 when I was on my way back to England from the Far East. Passing through Boston, I telephoned Denny-Brown. He invited me to stay with him, and I gave a lecture to his students on the psychological experiences of shipwreck survivors. He was a charming host, and we spent some time together happily rummaging through second-hand book shops, where I found some volumes to add to my growing collection dealing with The French Second Empire.

Denny-Brown joined the British Army. Commissioned in the Royal Army Medical Corps, he was posted to St. Hughes Hospital for Head Injuries at Oxford, which was presided over by Hugh Cairns and C.P. Symonds.

He returned to Boston for a time, but in 1945 the British Army recalled him and sent him to Poona in India as a Consultant in Neurology, with the rank of Brigadier. He succeeded Hugh Garland and Douglas McAlpine there.

When Denny-Brown returned to Boston after the war, he was appointed to the James Jackson Putnam Chair of Neurology. His numerous contributions to our discipline are well known and have been admirably described in Dr. Foley's detailed obituary of him.

After the war, I met him from time to time at Congresses and symposia, and I thought he showed the effects of his dedicated long hours of concentrated hard work.

Nevertheless, his published work was prolific, and extended over a wide neurological field. Like the admirable Crichton,

Denny-Brown tackled almost every aspect of neurology apart from psychiatry, psychology and philosophy. He wrote one paper on higher nervous activity in which he was bold enough to hypothesize an entity, which he called "morphosynthesis". As Ben Jonson wrote, "A man coins a new word not without peril, and less fruit, for if it happens to be received, the praise is but moderate; if refused, the scorn is assured."

He was not a great communicator on paper, and once had a postcard from F.M.R. Walshe which read, "Dear Denny, I see you have a paper in *Brain*. When is the English version coming out?".

Like Sherrington, he was at his best not when lecturing but when teaching students, and many British postgraduates elected to spend a year with him in Boston, rather than in France or Germany.

Retirement simply meant a concentration of effort. He had access to the New England Primate Center at Southborough, Massachusetts, and there he pursued his researches. Unhampered by the claims of a practising physician, he lived securely within the sanctity of Academe, at Harvard and Yale. But, as Dylan Thomas said, "he was no gray and tepid don, smelling of water biscuits". Away from his monkeys he was a jolly and generous companion, holding up bravely against the tribulations of a slow-advancing fatal illness.

One obituarist described Denny-Brown as "the dominating figure in neurology in the middle of the 20th century". I think this is an over-statement, but I believe he would have been a very great clinician if he had resisted the lure of experimental curiosity.

My personal knowledge of Denny-Brown's work is pre-war. By the 1930s his foot was firmly on the professional ladder and he was set for a private practice in neurology. But it was the wrong ladder for him. It was already clear that his heart was not in hospital wards, and he seemed more at ease and happier in the laboratory. He did not apply his physiology to the clinic, as Walshe had done. It was no surprise that he preferred to take up a Rockefeller scholarship at Yale, and that, mixing with men from other academic circles, he was tempted by a Chair at Harvard.

Obviously, London's loss was very much Harvard's gain. The facilities then may not have been as attractive as in other universities, but the prestige was considerable and the primates were there in profusion. It is apparent from the students who worked with him and who later became eminent in their own right, that Denny had something to offer which was stimulating and rare. His many contributions to the literature were an eloquent witness of his continuing dedication to neurology.

It is of interest that one obituarist said that of all his writing Denny-Brown was most proud of his assemblage of the works of Charles Sherrington; that the honour which most touched him was his honorary fellowship of Magdalen College; and that his happiest years were those spent among the primates after his retirement.

I retain a fond memory of a film made by Graeme Robertson when he was visiting Boston. He, Denny and Denny's small boys were on a wind-swept hill outside the city, flying kites. They were not altogether successful, but they were having a marvellous time. Neurology was a long way off that day.

1897–1971
Raymond Garcin

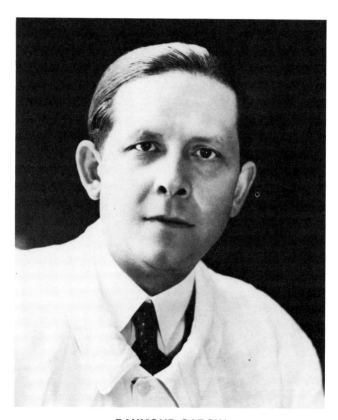

RAYMOND GARCIN

I knew Raymond Garcin so well and for so long that it is hard to put my memories into any logical order. "It is very strange to think back like this, although, come to think of it there is no fence or hedge around Time that has gone. You can go back and have what you like if you remember it well enough." The words are those of Richard Llewellyn, and I find them appropriate. For example, it is difficult for me to establish precisely when and in what circumstances we met. I believe the occasion was in March 1928, when I first went to Paris. I had been given a letter of introduction to the all-powerful Professor Georges Guillain who occupied the Charcot Chair of Neurology. At first sight he seemed a taciturn figure, and he surprised me by his extreme kindness. I stood at the periphery of a group of students around a patient's bed in the Salpêtrière, when Guillain insisted that I should come forward and witness some particularly unusual physical sign. After the ward round, Guillain came up to me and invited me to lunch the following day at his house. This was a courtesy and a compliment indeed.

He lived in a splendid but gloomy mansion in the Boulevard St. Germain. The luncheon was a family affair. I met Mme. Guillain, whose father, I believe, was Professor Chauffard. Then there were Professor Guillain's daughters, one of whom was married. I was introduced to her husband, Dr. Raymond Garcin, a neurologist then working at the Hôtel Dieu.

Garcin was at that time 31 years of age. He impressed me as a man of exceptional charm and intelligence, and likely to go far in his profession.

Over the next 40 years I got to know him well. His great modesty concealed the success he was continually achieving as he mounted the ladder of his career. Only gradually did I realise the intellectual status of my friend. Gold medallist among the internists of the year, he received wide recognition with his doctoral thesis, in which he described the case of a patient who had a paralysis of all the cranial nerves on one side. This rare phenomenon immediately received the name of the Raymond Garcin syndrome.

His subsequent career was spectacular. In 1953 he was accorded the Chair of Pathology and General Therapeutics, with a service at the Salpêtrière. This gave him the opportunity to display his astonishing ability as an exponent of clinical neurology. He was, I believe, the most popular teacher of neurology in Paris.

His clinical examination of a patient was carried out with extreme courtesy and gentleness, while at the same time it was most thorough. His technique has been likened to a work of art, by way of its precision, punctiliousness, clarity and elegance. There was little that escaped his scrutiny. Garcin never indulged in the habit—so common in European physicians—of pinching the cheeks of young lady patients, as a gesture of benevolence.

His students were unlikely to forget his running comments, for they were didactic and convincing. As long ago as 1902, William Gowers had emphasized the importance of repetition in conveying a message in neurology. ". . . a teacher who hesitates to repeat shrinks from his most important duty, and a learner who dislikes to hear the same thing twice over, lacks his most essential acquisition." Garcin went even further. He had a technique all of his own, believing in the dictum that "when I say a thing three times, it is so". He therefore triplicated his remarks. As Hilaire Belloc wrote: "First I tell them what I am going to say; then I say it; and afterwards I tell them what it is that I've just said." This verbal mannerism, be it noted, was confined to his teaching, and did not obtrude into his conversation.

Needless to say, he was held in particularly high esteem by his students. As Dr. Moya de Gonzalez of Madrid tells us, he had many disciples from Spain, Portugal and Latin America. On at least one occasion such pupils organised a dinner party to honour him and his wife.

During the Second World War I often wondered how my good friends in France and Holland were faring. It was a question that was never asked when the war had finished. Garcin was one of the few who spoke of the time when Paris was occupied. He told me that not once during the Occupation did he have occasion to speak to a German. Not so one of his sons. Garcin chuckled as he told me that his little boy, aged about 10, was stopped in the street by a soldier who enquired of him the way to some place. "I pointed in the opposite direction, daddy", he triumphantly told his father.

In 1959 the Charcot Chair of Neurology became vacant, and neurologists outside the bazaar of academic politics of Paris imagined that Garcin would be appointed. But that was not so. Garcin, however, was given a personal Chair of Clinical Neurology, and many structural alterations were made to his Department in the Pavilion Mazarin at the Salpêtrière. A daïs was erected at one end of the hall to afford the audience a better view of what the Professor was doing. This was an opportunity for his students to present him with an ecclesiastical *prie-dieu,* which enabled him to elicit and demonstrate his patient's ankle-jerks with greater *éclat.*

The catalogue of his contributions to neurology is bulky. Working as a young man in conjunction with Rademaker, he studied the loss of static adaptation. Later, he showed particular interest in the thalamus and in the cerebellum. He wrote a monograph upon "Les Ataxies". Viscosity of eye-movements intrigued him. He wrote upon the automatic blinking of the eyelids provoked by a threatening gesture, and he showed that this reflex could disappear after cortico-subcortical lesions even though there was no hemianopia.

Garcin's name will be remembered for his demonstration of *la main creuse* or the hollow hand. This, he regarded as the most delicate manual sign of an early pyramidal affection. It is shown when the patient holds up his hand and spreads his fingers as far as he can. Slowly the first metacarpal contracts in adduction. The thenar eminence becomes prominent and a crescentic crease forms in the palm. There is also a *main creuse tonique* which patients with chorea or with athetosis show promptly on separating the fingers, without the delay that characterises the classical *main creuse parétique*.

Garcin's command of English was incomplete. Whenever he came to lecture at the National Hospital, he elected to speak in French. I remember on one occasion volunteering to translate his words into English, paragraph by paragraph. The lecturer proceeded *accelerando, allegretto, con brio*. As his pace increased so did my difficulties, and his talk ended with a burst of laughter from the audience.

Apart from his neurological achievements, Raymond Garcin is remembered by me on two important counts—his conspicuous and wholly genuine courtesy, and his friendliness. I doubt whether anyone, anywhere, ever bore against him a trace of enmity or even ill-will. Once only did I see him angry, but he remained calm and restrained. He was deeply attached to his family—his charming wife, his daughter and three sons. Then, after an interval, came a fourth boy, whom he delighted to designate his "Benjamin". Dinner at the Garcins' was always a delightful family occasion, with father-in-law, Professor Guillain, frequently present. Sometimes there would be other guests, like Dr. Paul Guilly and his wife.

Dr. and Mme. Garcin were hospitable in the extreme. The fact that on my visits to Paris I was often in the company of Fergus Ferguson and Philip Cloake did not restrain his welcome. He delighted in referring to us as *les trois mousquétaires*. If Garcin was the perfect host at these dinners, he was also an ideal guest. On one of those rare occasions when it was possible to welcome a visitor to my own home and accommodate him, Garcin was courtly, appreciative and amusing.

Raymond Garcin was rather short and stocky, clean-shaven, with abundant jet-black hair. He was slightly barrel-chested and stooped a little. His expression was genial, almost boyish. By modern standards he smoked too much, his preference being for Gauloise cigarettes. His colleagues remarked that he spoke with a faint "accent of the islands"—presumably the product of his being born at Basse-Point, Martinique, and educated in its principal town, Fort-de-France.

For that matter, I was once informed that not one of the neurological giants of Paris was free from traces of a provincial accent of one kind or another. No doubt Garcin's Caribbean origins also explained his pleasant habit of serving rum as an aperitif before dinner.

I have long observed that the medical élite then in Paris seemed to rely upon taxis or chauffeur-driven limousines for transport across the city. Comparatively late in his professional career, Garcin surprised us all by buying a car—an extremely small one—in which he ventured out into the streets of Paris. I was one of his pioneer passengers. The experience was, to me, most alarming, but Garcin never for a moment betrayed anxiety or hesitation. He chatted to me gaily throughout the perilous expedition.

Once when in Paris, I learned that one of the Communists who had been accused of setting fire to the Reichstag in 1933, had sustained a stroke and was in a private hospital under the care of Professor Garcin. Some days later I went to dine with him. He was not in his usual bubbling spirits, but seemed *distrait*. I asked how was his notorious patient. "I don't know" was his reply. "When I went to pay my routine visit this afternoon I found his bed empty. He had gone." Apparently a number of men had entered the nursing home, taken the patient out of bed, and conveyed him by car to a waiting aircraft bound for Moscow. Garcin had not been notified, and he never heard another thing about the patient.

Some years later, exactly the same experience happened to me with a Russian patient in London.

Among the many distinctions which were accorded to Garcin was high office in the Legion of Honour, membership of the

Académie Nationale de Médecine, and the coveted Max Nonne gold medal of the German neurological society. He had the unusual distinction of being an honorary Fellow of the Royal College of Physicians of London; he was also an honorary Fellow of the Royal Society of Medicine.

Every August, Garcin and his family would leave Paris for their country property in Normandy. There he would write, relax and indulge in his hobby of landscape painting in water colours, one of which he gave to me. It was in this Normandy village that Raymond Garcin died on 27th February 1971, after some months of ill-health and great sorrow over the tragic death of his wife shortly before. His burial was a quiet one, in the local church.

Our French colleagues put us to shame when it comes to delivering an oration or tribute. This is demonstrated by the anonymous obituarist in the *Revue Neurologique* . . . "Raymond Garcin: loved by so many, respected by all. For one third of a century, my dear friend. Controlling my emotion, may I depict him to you as though he were still with us, living among his family, his patients and his confrères at the Société de Neurologie which he had served for so long? Even now we can imagine him joining us in our amphitheatre, entering by that door on the right, and slowly descending the stairs, ponderous and slightly stooping, his features noble and his eyes gentle, clasping in friendship hands stretched out to him, before finally taking his place in the front row with all the modesty of a truly great man surrounded by his beloved pupils and ardent admirers".

1878–1965
Kurt Goldstein

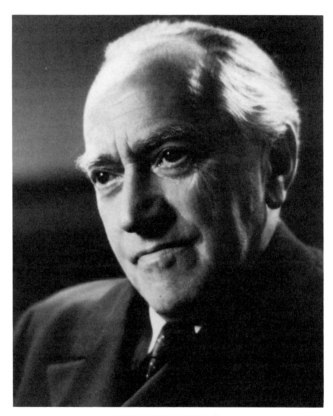

KURT GOLDSTEIN

From Critchley, M: *Parietal Lobes.* Edward Arnold, London, 1953.

B ecause of my interest in aphasiology—as I termed it— and in disorders of higher nervous activity as well as in the processes of ageing, I had long been aware of the work of Kurt Goldstein. Henry Head, in his monograph on *Aphasia and Kindred Disorders of Speech* (1926), had criticized many of the ideas that had been held regarding the nature and mechanism of language disorders. Unlike the materialists and localizationist "Diagram-makers", Hughlings Jackson had been accorded high praise, as had writers such as von Monakow, von Woerkom, Pick and Goldstein.

In addition to his work on aphasia, Goldstein had drawn attention to certain behavioural changes which were apt to follow brain-injury, additional to any speech-disorder that might be present. From the experience of a large series of brain-damaged soldiers, he recognised a fundamental alteration in cerebral activity reducing the patient's conduct to a more primitive level.

This is not the place for a detailed recapitulation of the interesting views expressed by Goldstein, and such co-workers of his as Scheerer. Elsewhere I have summarized some of his important views (*Parietal Lobes,* London: Arnold, 1953). If the brain-injured patient, or the "organism" to use Goldstein's terminology, is confronted with tasks that are within his capacity, he will perform them in a harmonious, orderly fashion. Faced, however, with an assignment with which he cannot readily cope, he is liable to betray a "catastrophic reaction"—annoyance, anger, tears, for example. His life-style becomes restricted to an environment or milieu that is undemanding. Many of the seemingly perplexing patterns of behaviour are, in fact, the expression of the sick man's flight from the risk of a catastrophic reaction. To achieve an acceptable milieu, various devices may be adopted, such as self-exclusion; avoidance of company; restless over-activity; a cloak of indifference; excessive orderliness; or a meticulous adherence to a time-schedule. The patients are not aware of their altered personalities, or even of the nature and extent of their disabilities. The more severe the defect in "instrumentalities" (motor, sensory, visual, verbal), the greater the adjustment. Goldstein formulated a number of types of disintegration which follow neurological lesions: (1) the threshold of excitation rises, so that the rate of performance becomes slower; (2) once excitation has been achieved, it continues for an undue length of time (hence the phenomenon of perseveration); (3) various factors influence the patient overmuch resulting either in distractibility, or in the opposite state of being "stimulus-bound"; and (4) constant difficulty in distinguishing essentials from non-essentials, or, in the Gestalt metaphor, "figure" from "ground".

Perhaps to Goldstein the most important postulate was that the brain-injured person loses the ability to assume a "categorical attitude". In other words, he can no longer emerge from an elementary, passive type of concrete behaviour. This alteration in comportment is one which is reflected in numerous ways in his daily life, in his speech, and in his response to test procedures.

The foregoing remarks comprise a mere outline of Goldstein's remarkable interpretation of man's reaction to brain injury. Trauma is by no means the sole determinant in such circumstances. The same difficulties with categorical behaviour apply to patients with brain tumour, cerebral arteriopathy, the dementias, and even senility.

Goldstein's philosophy appeared upon the neuropsychiatric scene like a blast of fresh air, dispelling some of the dust of atomistic thinking, making clear much of what had been obscure, and offering prospects of mental rehabilitation. Neurological sticklers may, of course, argue that there is a paucity of statistical evidence as well as a lack of data of a personal and environmental kind, including sex, age, race, intelligence and educational status.

Objective evidence of impaired categorical attitude is usually demonstrated by a "sorting test", the best known having been devised by Weigl, a pupil of Goldstein. Along with Scheerer in 1941, Goldstein produced a battery of such testing techniques which was popular for a time, but, as the psychologist Aaron Smith pointed out in 1975, "because of the lack of normative data and clinical estimates rather than objective quantative scoring procedures, its earlier popularity has waned."

Who was this erudite expositor? I wondered how I could meet him.

He had been born in Germany, I learned, in the Upper Silesian town of Kattowitz (now in Poland and known as Katowice). Having trained in Breslau (now Wroclaw), where Otfried Foerster was five years his senior, he proceeded to Berlin, Heidelberg and Frankfurt, under such teachers as Carl Wernicke and Ludwig Edinger. By an odd quirk of fate, many years later Goldstein was to examine the morphology of Edinger's brain and, in association with Walter Riese, publish a monograph on the subject. At that time, there was a vogue for studying *Elitegehirnen,* which led to a series of examinations of the brains of eminent scientists and musicians.

In the First World War, Goldstein had been in charge of the institute in Frankfurt for Research into Brain Injuries. There he worked in association with Gelb, a Gestaltist. Many papers resulted from their cooperation. Of particular importance was a monograph dealing with a patient named Schneider, who was to become a legendary figure. I shall refer to it later.

It is doubtful whether Goldsteinian doctrines ever became wholly absorbed within the corpus of neurological thought and teaching, but his ideas were never specifically rejected. Perhaps they were ignored—the unkindest cut of all. The words of Oscar Wilde may give a clue: "There are works which wait and which one does not understand for a long time; the reason is that they bring answers to questions which have not yet been raised; for the question often arrives a terribly long time after the answer."

Goldstein's reputation at Frankfurt was considerable, and in 1930 there were plans to tempt him to Berlin to take charge of a new research institute. He accepted, with the proviso that he would also keep in close touch with Frankfurt. In January 1933, however, with the onset of the Nazi regime, the programme was cancelled. Goldstein was jailed for a short time. He was released on condition that he left Germany. Supported by the Rockefeller Foundation, he lived for a year in Amsterdam, a sojourn that gave him the opportunity to write *The Organism*. In 1935 he went to New York, where he was afforded a Professorship of Clinical Neurology at Columbia.

Then came an invitation from Harvard to deliver the William James lectures. So successful were they that he was offered a five-year Professorship at Tufts University. Here he was invited to teach undergraduates, but his thoughts were perhaps too abstruse and his command of English was possibly not fluent enough for him to attain popularity among students. As Goethe put it: *Hyposthesen sind Wiegenlieder womit der Lehrer seine Schüler einlüllt.* (Theories are the lullabies wherewith the teacher lulls his pupils to sleep.) The average undergraduate was not on the same wavelength, and his teaching was caviare to the general. Among older and more serious students of philosophy and of psychology, he was extremely popular.

After that period he had reached the age of retirement, and he returned to New York. Goldstein engaged in private practice and taught at the City Hospital. He also paid a weekly visit to Brandeis University at Waltham, Massachusetts.

I first met Goldstein in New York in 1952, in the company of Israel Wechsler. Whenever we met after that, it was usually within the precincts of Mount Sinai Hospital, where he had been made welcome by Israel Wechsler and Morris Bender.

Goldstein had a gentle, sad face, and was most courteous and congenial in demeanour. I had many opportunities of talking with him during the annual meetings of the American Neurological Association which I attended. He told me of his experiences with Edinger, Oppenheim, Wernicke and other giants of German neurology. It was obvious that we shared interests that lay a little outside the commonplace activities of the clinic. He gave me a copy of the English edition of his monograph *The Organism*. Whenever I lectured in New York, Goldstein was present. His contributions to the discussion were shrewd and friendly.

In 1953 I heard that he would be passing through London on his way to Frankfurt, and I immediately invited him to lecture at the National Hospital. He agreed, and on that occasion the lecture theatre was fuller than I had seen it before or since. The address was brilliantly developed, and well received. Afterwards I arranged a small dinner party for Professor and Mrs. Goldstein at the Connaught Hotel, and also invited F.M.R. Walshe, Dr. and Mrs. Eric Strauss and Dr. and Mrs. Swithin Meadows.

The following day Professor Goldstein came to my consulting rooms and I gave him a copy of my book *The Parietal Lobes*. I mentioned that his famous patient, Schneider, had also been examined by several neurologists besides himself, in particular by Professor Bay, and that they had queried some of Goldstein's opinions as to the nature of the case. Goldstein was surprised, and seemed rather put out. He told me that when he reached Frankfurt, he would try to contact his old patient. Whether he already knew about these differing opinions, I am not sure.

Shortly afterwards, a postcard arrived from Goldstein in Germany to say that he had seen Schneider and that everything was the same as he had said. It is now necessary to go back in time.

During the First World War there came under the care of Kurt Goldstein at the Frankfurt Brain Institute, a soldier aged 24 who had received severe injuries to the occipital region of the skull. A complicated clinical picture developed with defects principally in vision. In association with Gelb, Goldstein studied the patient with extreme thoroughness, and they came to the conclusion that Schn. (or Schneider, to give him his actual name) was a case of that rare condition, Lissauer's apperceptive mind-blindness. Later, Goldstein wrote that he would prefer to regard the diagnosis not so much as an agnosia as a *Gestaltblindheit* . . . "a disturbance of visual recognition due to a defect in the perceptual sphere concerning the step of gestalt formation." Gelb and Goldstein published their account of Schn. in 1918 in an article comprising 171 pages of the *Z.N.P.*, vol. 41.

When Goldstein had to leave Germany, it was inevitable that the patient should come under the care of other neurologists, some of whom published their findings. Others, like Russell Brain (*Brain*, 1941, vol. 64), for example, took issue with Goldstein on theoretical grounds without having seen the patient. Russell Brain was a serious thinker and the mildest of men, but his paper angered Goldstein and he published a rather tart reply in the *J.N.M.D.*, 1943:98.

Kleist (1922) regarded the diagnosis as one of a perceptive disability, not agnosia. Poppelreuter (1923) rejected the idea of mind-blindness and looked upon the patient as a victim of "a peculiar visual defect". Pötzl accepted Goldstein and Gelb's conclusions but with some reservations. Both Quensel (1931) and Lange (1936) threw doubt upon the reliability of much of Schn.'s evidence. Writing from America in 1943, Goldstein stoutly defended his original concept.

Schneider was discharged from the Army on a 70% disability pension. Leaving hospital, he married and in 1931 opened a food shop. In 1943 he sold the business and then came under the care of Professor E. Bay. Jointly with O. Lauenstein and P. Cibis, Bay published a full account of their findings in the case of Schneider in *Psych. Neur. Med. Psychol.*, 1949:1. They found a considerable visual defect, in spite of which the patient comported himself normally in everyday life. The authors regarded Schneider as being unreliable, contradictory and often inaccurate in his statements. They hinted that the complicated visual picture had developed only after years of repeated

psychological examinations. The patient was unusually accom-
modating and eager to help. After long training, he had attained
a virtuosity which he still displayed 20 years later (1949).

In the same year, the case was discussed by R. Jung, his
examination of the patient having taken place in 1942. He felt
sure that many of Schn.'s defects were the product of suggestion,
and of examinations that had been too detailed and too many.
Jung commented that had the patient originally been examined
by a psychotherapist (instead of by a brain pathologist and a
gestalt psychologist), there might have been both a different
interpretation and a different outcome.

In 1952 I learned that Schneider was acting as Bürgermeister
of a small town in South Germany. In December of that year,
however, Professor Leonhard told me that Schneider had
resigned from his post, and that he was now working in the
ticket-office of a small railway station.

These details I quoted in *Parietal Lobes*. I merely reported
the observations without making any comment or expression
of opinion. Indeed, I had no personal views, never having seen
the patient. At the same time, I knew Russell Brain, Jung and
Bay quite well and held all three in high regard. But, as the
Ancient Greeks said, "Mountain will not mingle with mountain".

Then followed an interesting correspondence. First came the
postcard already referred to, in which Goldstein told me he
had met Schneider and that his condition was as he had
previously described.

A letter dated 9th August 1953 followed, from Switzerland:
". . . I want to tell you further that I have seen the patient
Schneider in Frankfurt. He is in a very good general condition
but in all respects we have described exactly the same as before,
he has only learned still more than before to compensate by
roundabout ways—the same we have described before—the
incapacities which are unchanged. It is unbelievable how somewhat [sic] (? someone) could assume that he tried to deceive—
what he absolutely is due to his defect unable as us shown [sic]
before. Therefore I am convinced that Bay's assertion is based

on lack of careful observations. Later more about! . . ." Unfortunately, I have no copies of my replies.

Whether Goldstein ever examined Schneider yet again is uncertain. He must have seriously pondered over the problem and re-read the diverse criticisms that had been made by various neurologists, because he wrote a detailed restatement of the problem, in German, from New York. His paper, entitled: "Bemerkungen zur Methodik der Untersuchung psychopathologischen Fälle—Im Anschluss an die Nachuntersuchung des 'seelenblinden' Patientin Schneider, mehrals 30 Jahre nach dem Auftraten der Störung" appeared in the *Monat. f. P. u. N.,* 1956:131. (Remarks upon the method of examination of psychopathological cases. In conclusion the follow-up examination of the "mind blind" patient, Schneider. More than 30 years after the onset of the lesion.)

Before the publication of this paper, I received a five-page typed letter, dated 15th July 1954, which distressed me. He must have re-read my remarks in *Parietal Lobes,* and was particularly upset because I had referred to the Schneider controversy. In addition, my evaluation of Goldsteinian conceptions in general, though highly laudatory, also contained a few mild animadversions that annoyed him.

Goldstein's complaints were threefold: (1) I had quoted (without comment, be it noted) the findings of several neurologists whose conclusions about Schneider had been at variance with his own: Professor Bay's contribution provoked his particular displeasure; (2) I had mentioned various weaknesses in Goldstein's main theory, namely the lack of scientific evaluation along statistical lines; and (3) I had omitted to give him credit for certain subtleties of clinical technique that he had described and recorded. As to Goldstein's third objection, my remarks were original and owed nothing to his work—of which I was unaware.

Goldstein ended his letter with these words: "Believe me, this letter is one of the most disagreeable things I did in my life. Maybe therefore I have postponed it so long. Even now I would like to throw it in the waste basket. But I estimate you so highly and we both Eva and I like you personally so much that I feel I have to do it, and to ask you why does one treat me so in general and particularly you! I do not think that this letter should disturb our friendship. Yours" [unsigned].

He wrote to me again on 7th August 1954, from Switzerland. The letter, which again was unsigned, was written by hand. Some parts were difficult to interpret, but I believe the following is the correct version: "Dear Dr. Critchley, . . . I'd like to add some words to the sentences in your book in relation to Schneider's *"work"*. He worked! As I have mentioned in my papers, that he worked in the workshop connected with the hospital and did very precise work. We could by very careful analysis show that what he did corresponded to his (? previous) capacities and he was able to do it in spite of his defects. He did so in a way *essentially different* from normals and only if we studied his *way of working* we could not be deceived in the judgement about abnormality even here.

This concerns the two results of Bay you mentioned. *First:* the latest news of this notorious patient is that at the present time he is a Bürgermeister in a small town in South Germany— I know that but my information about the situation made it absolutely clear that he had not to do anything what he could not do in spite of his defect and all things which he could not do his wife did for him. As he volunteered to tell us right away, when I spoke with him about. The same was the case when he worked various occasions before. *Why did not Bay try to find out what he did?* and used the story as an appreciation to our interpretation of the symptoms in general and his work. How could you bring the nonsense in your book, which the other author, the name I have forgotten, says: 'had the patient originally been examined by a psychotherapist instead by a brain pathologist and a gestalt psychologist then there might have been both a different interpretation and also a different outcome' (284 of your book). I really would like to understand what has gone on in your mind that you gave these men more credit than my investigations! which explained that the patient could behave in *this way to his defect!* August 7 1954. Switzerland" [unsigned].

Obviously I had unwittingly offended a man whose work I much admired and had repeatedly quoted to my students and colleagues. He was also someone I held in affection and respect.

Some great innovators and some very wise men are super-sensitive whenever their work is called in question, however gently. But, then, why should they not be umbrageous? Their genius entitles them to take pride in their achievements. As Dr. Johnson said: "Who am I to bandy words with my sovereign?".

I wrote a long reply to him, restating my high opinion of him personally and of his great contributions to neuropsychology. To mention in print that contrary opinions had been expressed upon the nature of the case Schneider was, I thought, only fair, and that I was not "taking sides" in the dispute. Professor Goldstein was, I hope and believe, mollified, to some extent at any rate.

On his 80th birthday I sent him a letter of congratulations, to which I received the following gracious note:

> New York Nov. 30 1958. I thank you dear Dr. Critchley. Your letter was a source of real joy for me. Your words gave me the good feeling that the relationship between you and us which we appreciated so much is unchanged, that it was solid enough not to be disturbed by some misunderstanding. So your letter was for me a real birthday present. Thank you Dr. Critchley. Mrs. Goldstein sends you best regards. Cordially yours, Kurt Goldstein. I appreciated very much the telegram from Queen Square Hospital.

Over the ensuing years, Professor Goldstein remained well and mentally vigorous. He continued to write, and he enjoyed the company of intellectual friends. But he realised he was tired and ageing. The blow struck in the summer of 1965, when he sustained an apoplexy. He remained conscious but he was hemiplegic and—what could be more cruel—aphasic. What a grim irony that one who had devoted so much of his life to a study of the nature of language and its dissolution, should be rendered speechless. Were there perhaps compensations of a sort? In his silent prison, was he vouchsafed a glimpse through its high windows of the broad acres of human communication? Maybe he was able to realise the answers to some of the philosophic and transcendental questions he had pondered for years. Mercifully, this ambiguous state in which he lay crippled, mute and incommunicable was relatively brief, and after three weeks he quietly died, aged 87.

* * * * * * *

And what of Schneider—victim of two wars, one of which was academic? If he is alive today he is 94 years of age. Professor Bay kindly informs me (October 1988) that, as far as he knows, no further neurological studies of him have been published, and that no record of any autopsy has yet appeared. It seems probable that he has died, unrecorded, a controversial figure to the end.

1898–1973
Fritz Grewel

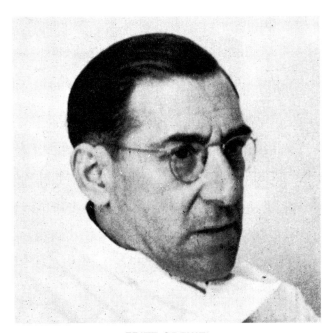

FRITZ GREWEL

From Critchley, M: *Aphasiology*, Edward Arnold, London, 1970.

M ore than 50 years ago, it became obvious that the study of aphasia would gain a great deal from the impact of linguistics, and vice versa. Before the discipline of psycholinguistics had come about, a few neurologists were beginning to draw upon what used to be called philology in the analysis of their patients who had sustained some affection of speech. Among this small group of pioneers was Fritz Grewel of Amsterdam.

He was a most erudite man. As the poet Cowper said: "Knowledge is proud that he has learned so much; Wisdom is humble that he knows no more?". But he was far too self-effacing, and he is now apt to be overlooked.

In 1951, Grewel had enumerated the various linguistic disturbances that aphasiacs may show. These included (1) lexical losses; (2) phonemic disturbances; (3) paraphonemia; (4) paraphasia; (5) agrammatism and paragrammatism; (6) disorders in the system of accents; and (7) defects in the non-verbal forms of communication.

An important paper was published by Grewel in 1957 in which he classified the various types of dysarthria encountered in clinical practice.

His many other published works indicated that we shared several interests in neurology besides aphasia—the punch-drunk syndrome in boxers; the Kleine-Levin syndrome; developmental dyslexia; parietal lobe symptomatology; and also "nonsense talk" both in Dutch and in English.

Even before the Second World War, I was fortunate enough to meet Grewel on my visits to Holland, and he entertained me to dinner at his house. His cultural and neurological lore were both broad and deep; I felt that I was in the presence of an exceptional man of great wisdom and yet simplicity. He had a gentleness of manner that reminded me of Goldstein, without the latter's over-sensitiveness.

Professionally speaking, he was a paediatric neuropsychiatrist. The Dutch, like the Greeks, have a name for it—orthopedagogics. In 1930, Grewel had been appointed head of the polyclinic for Child Psychiatry at the famous Wilhelmina Gasthuis in Amsterdam. In 1933, in association with Mulock Haver and Koekebakker, he organised a group dedicated to the mission of child protection.

His academic advance was distinguished. In 1954 he became lector (or reader) in Child Psychiatry; and in 1965 he was appointed to the Chair of Orthopedagogics within the Faculty of Social Sciences.

Dr. Grewel visited London to lecture at the National Hospital. He chose as his theme "Acalculia". His talk was highly impressive, and the paper was subsequently published in *Brain* (1952, vol. 75). Another version appears in the Vinken and Bruyn *Handbook of Clinical Neurology, vol. 4.* Grewel thoroughly explored this topic, and his work must surely be *le dernier cri*. His conclusion was that "in acalculia it is not a biological function, but a sociogenic learned behaviour or performance, a conditioned semiotic system, that has suffered."

We continued to correspond, and, whenever I visited Amsterdam, I called upon him. He and I would browse in the fine antiquarian bookshops that abound in that city.

Early in 1960 we met at a conference on the evolution of language which had been organised by the Swedish Werner-Gren Foundation. The meeting was held in the ancient Wartenstein Castle, situated near the small town of Gloggnitz midway between Vienna and Graz. Until recently it had been occupied by Russian troops. There were 16 participants, and the procedure was rather unusual. Each one of us was asked in advance to write an essay on the subject. The papers were printed and circulated before the meeting.

We were accommodated in the castle and foregathered in a large room, in the centre of which the 16 of us sat around a circular table. If there was a chairman, I cannot remember who it was.

As a group we were international, two members coming from the Netherlands, one each from Italy, Spain, Germany and England, and the rest from the United States of America. With three exceptions, all were academics. Some were quite young. Between us, we represented the disciplines of biology, anthropology, linguistics and semiotics; there was also one expert in the so-called dancing language of bees. The three non-academics were Grewel, a paediatric neuropsychiatrist; my old friend Subirana from Barcelona, a neurologist who specialised in sinistrality, ambidexterity and cerebral dominance; and myself.

It soon became evident that little rapport existed between the pedagogues and the clinicians. The former appeared self-assured and slightly aggressive. "Facts fled from them like frightened forest things", as Oscar Wilde said. Ideas were for them either jet black or dead white, and the conception of shades of grey was confined to Grewel, Subirana and me. Of course, the three of us were the only ones who worked among sick and distressed fellow creatures. One wondered how long it would be before these bold schoolmen sought relief or reassurance from one of the practising doctors they slightly despised.

In my contribution I suggested that in the phylogenetic trail linking animal communication to human language, a change had occurred at the point between the anthropoid apes and homo sapiens. This idea seemed shocking to at least one of the scientists; the others appeared uninterested.

Hours were spent debating the propriety of the term "symbol". On the whole, it was a word the academics disliked.

A day's rest was proclaimed half way through, and transport was arranged to take us to Vienna. The impact of mid-European culture was something that bewildered not a few of the party.

We took lunch at the famous Drei Huszaren restaurant, and in the evening were fortunate in securing seats at the Opera House. We heard Giordano's "André Chénier" conducted by Martinu, which was most impressive.

For the last evening, festivities were arranged. Special dishes were prepared for the dinner, and bottles of Kremser Wachtsberg were there in abundance. Tensions eased and conversation was freer, almost jolly. Even the men of Lagardo relaxed from extracting sunbeams out of cucumbers and attempting to convert ice into gunpowder. We "cried for madder music and stronger wine". Fritz Grewel actually burst into song, and we listened with enjoyment to his pleasing baritone voice.

The Werner-Gren symposium ended; the evolution of language remained as mysterious as ever. Possibly the sole outcome of the conference was an agreement, on the part of the academics, to outlaw the term "symbol".

Unfortunately I did not see Fritz Grewel again. He died in 1973. The departure of great men is "marked by footprints in the sands of time". He left footprints which are still detectable by those who are sensitive and sympathetic. "We see him as he moved, How modest, kindly, All accomplished, wise."

1886–1961
Sir Geoffrey Jefferson

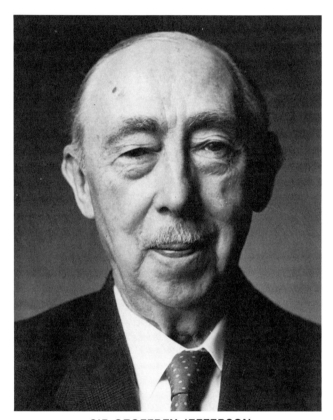

SIR GEOFFREY JEFFERSON

Courtesy of the Royal College of Physicians, London.

When one finds in a surgeon exquisite manipulative skill coupled with superlative intelligence and the mind of a philosopher, the product is exceptional. Geoffrey Jefferson was one such man. The Welsh have an axiom: "Gweddw crefft heb ai dawn", which roughly means "without inspiration, technical skill is sterile."[1] In that same vein, F.M.R. Walshe would sometimes irritably reproach a surgical colleague for displaying the triumph of technique over reason.

During my many visits to Manchester, where my good friend Fergus Ferguson was neurologist to the Royal Infirmary, I often met his neurosurgical colleague, Jefferson. Though 14 years younger, Ferguson had actually been on the staff for the same length of time as Jefferson, who had previously worked at the Salford Royal Hospital. Occasionally I heard him lecture, and sometimes I went to the operating theatre to watch him at work.

In those days, most of my contact with him was limited to chats in the ward side-room over cups of coffee when three or four of us were present. Our talk was largely neurological "shop", laced with gossip and a touch of scandal. Jefferson's comments were always shrewd and often witty. Unlike many neurosurgeons of that period, he was deeply interested in the science and art of neurology and even psychiatry. He had a great sense of fun, and his slow, deliberate conversation was often interrupted by a characteristic chuckle.

---

[1] Mr. Wyn Roberts, M.P., Secretary of State at The Welsh Office, kindly informs me that in this text, the key word is "gweddw", which generally means "widowed". The literal meaning is "widowed is a craft that is without talent".

In 1933, a few others and I decided to form a small, exclusive neurological club. We elected Wilfrid Harris as President, Gordon Holmes as Secretary and Kinnier Wilson as Treasurer. Seven years before, however, Jefferson had been instrumental in founding the Association of British Neurosurgeons—familiarly known to us as the Nutcrackers. By an odd chance, I happened to sit in on one of the business meetings held before the actual formation of their Association. Jefferson was obviously the driving force, and I remember the manner in which he coped with all who doubted or who were half-hearted. The seniority of some of those present did not inhibit him in any way.

At that time I did not know much about Jefferson's background, and, in particular, was unaware that early in the First World War he had served in an Anglo-Russian Hospital organised by Herbert Waterlow. I regret not having talked to him about it, for in my youth it had been my romantic idea to join the Russian air force. I had taken evening classes in Russian in my last year at school and during my first year as a medical student for that very purpose. Unfortunately for my plans, the Revolution broke out in October 1917, and my military service did not take me to Russia. I would have liked to quiz Jefferson about his experiences in Petrograd, a city which I came to know later.

In 1933 Jefferson was invited to join the staff of the National Hospital in London. This step was not taken without considerable argument between the diehard members of the staff and the younger ones who realised that neurosurgery at Queen Square was in the doldrums. But, by this time, Jefferson was already in charge of a highly professional department of neurosurgery. He elected to carry on with his academic duties in Manchester and to live in that city, but to visit London roughly every two weeks. He would see patients who were referred to him and, if necessary, operate.

We Londoners discovered what his colleagues in Manchester

had long known. He had absolutely no sense of time, and it did not worry him.

Some evenings I would see him in the Athenaeum Club in a state of uncertainty as to whether to dine there, whether to spend the night in London, or whether to return to Manchester. He was bemused but calm and detached. On the other hand, his disorientation caused a considerable strain on the surgical theatre staff, the resident housemen, the anaesthetists and, above all, the patients.

For example, it might be arranged over the telephone that Jefferson would operate at, say, 10 a.m. on Thursday. The patient would be prepared for surgery and was ready to face the ordeal. He might even be in the anaesthetic room. Jefferson might not appear until the following day, without comment or explanation, quite unperturbed. His quiet charm and uncon-cern disarmed the frustrated staff. What the bewildered pa-tient's feelings were, can only be surmised.

Cushing was a slow operator; so was Halsted; so was Leriche. Geoffrey Jefferson must surely have out-dallied them all. He would take many hours to carry out a straightforward brain operation that would have taken his colleague Wylie McKissock an hour, and Percy Sargent 45 minutes. In the middle of an operation Jefferson might pause, wander out into an anteroom, sit down, and perhaps smoke a cigarette and drink a cup of coffee. Refreshed, he would scrub up again and resume his surgery.

Jefferson's appointment to the staff of the National Hospital marked the pinnacle of Cushing's influence on British neuro-surgery. Jefferson shared the role of disciple with two other surgeons—Norman Dott of Edinburgh and Hugh Cairns of the London Hospital. In their missionary zeal, both became so dictatorial that medical neurologists often found it difficult to work with them. Dott became a sick man, but he controlled his surgical department with fierce authority from his bed in the Royal Infirmary. Cairns was appointed to the National Hospital at the same time as Jefferson, but while the latter visited infrequently and largely unpredictably, Cairns did not turn up at all. His demands as to staff and equipment were unacceptable to the National Hospital. Later he left London for the Nuffield Chair of Surgery at Oxford. When the war came in 1939 and Brigadier Hugh Cairns worked at the Oxford Head Injuries Unit, he met his match in his opposite number, Air Vice-Marshal C.P. Symonds.

Of the three avant-garde crusaders in British neurosurgery, Jefferson was the cleverest, the most reasonable, the one most interested in neuroscience, and the one who was most ready to compromise. He had a mischievous charm, which he deliberately used to achieve his aims. His influence upon British neurosurgery was paramount. He was looked up to as a Nestor, weighty in counsel and high in distinction.

Penfield wrote of Jefferson as "a man of intriguing whimsical philosophies. He was a surgeon who schooled himself in neurology by direct observation of the patient after the manner of Hughlings Jackson."

Whatever the nature of his apprenticeship, Jefferson did not belong to that category so castigated by F.M.R. Walshe in 1931, when he wrote: "The young neurosurgeon expects with no preliminary training to spring Minerva-like from the head of Harvey Cushing, fully armed and with nothing to learn after a single year's gestation". Walshe certainly did not have Jefferson in mind, for he held him in the highest esteem.

Jefferson was, of course, a Fellow of the Royal College of Surgeons. When later he was honoured by being elected an honorary Fellow of the Royal College of Physicians, I sent him a telegram: "Congratulations. Twice the Fellow you used to be". He replied: "You should have said 'three times'. I have also been made a Fellow of the Royal Society". That was indeed a great honour, one rarely accorded to a practising clinician.

Jefferson received many honorary doctorates, and he delivered numerous "named" lectures. He wrote a large number of papers dealing with a variety of neurosurgical topics. He did not publish any imposing monograph, though in 1960 a collection of selected papers was issued by Pitman Medical Books. His earliest contributions to the literature were upon morphological subjects reflecting his work under the supervision of Professor Elliot Smith, the world-famed anatomist.

Among the many important committees of which he was a member, was the Medical Research Council. His colleague and fellow member, Sir Douglas Black, wrote that Jefferson "understood everything except the passage of time".

Geoffrey's portrait was painted by Sir Gerald Kelly and was exhibited in the Royal Academy. It now hangs in the Royal College of Surgeons, Lincoln's Inn.

During the Second World War, Jefferson occupied the important post of Consultant Adviser in Neurosurgery to the Ministry of Health and Pensions. This office gave him great authority to set up centres of excellence, and to ensure that appropriate cases were sent to appropriate units without delay.

Although he was born in Rochdale, County Durham, Jefferson was a Mancunian by adoption. He was educated at the prestigious Manchester Grammar School, and received his medical training at the local university. Manchester is renowned for the outstanding figures in art, literature, music and medicine who were born or who worked there. How true was the statement Disraeli made almost 150 years ago ... "rightly understood, Manchester is as great a human exploit as Athens".

Jefferson died on 29th January 1961 leaving two sons, one a neurologist at Birmingham, the other a neurosurgeon at Sheffield.

Paraphrasing Oscar Wilde, neurosurgery has been defined as the pursuit of the incurable by the irrepressible. Jefferson certainly allowed no obstacles to restrain his intelligence from wandering widely for the benefit of many. Were he living today, he would be regarded as conservative and all-knowing. Jefferson was the neurosurgeon's surgeon, whose influence upon the status of his discipline in Great Britain has been second only to Victor Horsley. *Molto egli opro col senno e con la mano.* Tasso. (Great were his exploits both in brain and hand.)

1884–1952
Foster Kennedy

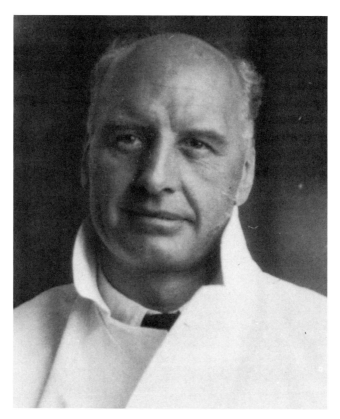

FOSTER KENNEDY

Courtesy of Lady Butterfield.

Good fairies were surely present at the birth of Foster Kennedy in Belfast on 7th February 1884. His was a much respected family comprising many academics. That very great soldier, Field Marshal Sir John Dill, was his cousin. Foster Kennedy was bestowed with intelligence, courage and great charm. The last-named quality was genuine, as evidenced by his considerable kindness and humanity. Such gifts were allied to that subtle endowment, the luck of the Irish.

Foster Kennedy qualified in medicine at Queen's College, Belfast, at the earliest possible age of 21. Already he had mapped out the course of his career: his ambition was to be a neurologist and to train in London. He secured a letter of introduction to Purves Stewart, who in turn commended him to Victor Horsley. Foster Kennedy wasted no time but tracked Horsley down to the National Hospital, Queen Square, where he was doing a ward round. Far from being annoyed by this intrusion, Horsley was impressed, and invited Foster to accompany him. He then went out of his way to give him advice, saying he should aim at obtaining a post as House Physician at the National Hospital. Should no vacancy occur then or in the near future, he should apply to be a Clinical Assistant to one of the honorary staff.

Actually there was such a vacancy, and Foster was elected to the resident medical staff, without having served the usual six, twelve or eighteen months in general medicine. At that time, there were two House Physicians, and Foster Kennedy's senior colleague was Kinnier Wilson. When Wilson was appointed Medical Registrar, Kennedy became the senior resident, his junior colleague being H.R. Prentice.

Kennedy was a resident for four years, and was probably Gowers' last house physician. From the many letters which Kennedy wrote to his fiancée, Miss Isabel McCann,[2] we learn that Gowers was in poor health and possibly failing in intellectual drive, and he retired prematurely. By then Gowers was, in all likelihood, increasingly difficult and cantankerous. Horsley seems to have been the chief who took the greatest interest in Foster Kennedy.

At the end of his four-year apprenticeship, Foster Kennedy looked around for a neurological appointment as a consultant, but in vain. Horsley and even Gowers did their best on his behalf, but without success. The fact that he was not a member of the Royal College of Physicians may have been a handicap. Suddenly, out of the blue, came an offer from America. In New York, three physicians, Pearce Bailey, Joseph Collins and Joseph Fraenkel, were in the throes of establishing a Neurological Institute. Premises were found in East 67th Street and the Institute was opened in December, 1909. Charles Elsberg was appointed surgeon in attendance. Kennedy was offered the post of Chief of Staff with a salary equivalent to £80 a year, and with a right to practice as soon as he had passed the examination all foreign doctors had to take.

In August 1910, Ramsay Hunt resigned his post as Assistant to Charles Dana, who occupied the Chair of Neurology at Cornell University. Dr. Dana asked Dr. Fraenkel whether Kennedy could take Ramsay Hunt's place. This was agreed.

Foster Kennedy rented an office at 52 West 53rd Street, being then 26 years of age. In September 1912, his fiancée left England for America and they married.

The year 1911 had seen the publication of his series of five cases where the diagnosis of a subfrontal brain tumour was made on the basis of unilateral optic atrophy with papilledema in the other eye (*Am. J. Med. Sci.*, vol. 142; *J. Nerv. Ment. Dis.*,

---

[2] This correspondence has been privately printed by his daughter, Lady Butterfield, under the title, *The Making of a Neurologist*, 1981.

vol. 38). His first case had been seen two years previously, when he was House Physician to Gowers, who published a paper on the subject (*Lancet*, 1909). The phenomenon has become known as the Foster Kennedy syndrome, and rightly so. His papers in 1911 went far to establish his reputation in New York.

Dana retired in 1919 and Foster Kennedy succeeded him as Professor of Neurology, with beds at Bellevue Hospital.

Meanwhile, he was building up a profitable private practice. His progress was assisted by Dana, who referred many patients to him.

When the first World War began in 1914, Foster Kennedy did not hesitate but left New York and joined the Royal Army Medical Corps as a six-month volunteer with the rank of Lieutenant. He and two others were instrumental in setting up a hospital in France. Difficulties arose initially in finding a suitable site, but eventually the French Government gave them a disused monastery in the village of Ris-Orangis. Mrs. Foster Kennedy followed her husband and worked in the hospital kitchens.

Kennedy was naturally anxious to be working as a neurologist, but there was only one such consultant in the British Army, namely Gordon Holmes. Kennedy dealt with acute battle casualties. Gradually his special experience was utilised, and his opinion was increasingly sought about head injuries and also cases of so-called "shell-shock". At the end of six months as a volunteer, Kennedy elected to stay on in France and was promoted to the rank of Captain. Mrs. Kennedy had to leave war work in France. For his services to the French Army, Foster was appointed Chevalier of the Legion of Honour.

Some, but not all, of the foregoing was known to me before I met him. As an aphasiologist, I was familiar with his interesting notion of "stock-brainedness" as a factor in the aetiology of "crossed-aphasia" (*Am. J. Med. Sci.*, 1916, vol. 152). I had also read with considerable interest his description of a temporary loss of artistic ability as the result of cranial trauma. This was a case report he had quoted in an address given to the New

York Academy of Medicine in 1936, entitled "The Organic Background of Mind". The patient was an honours student at a school of art. She had fallen and struck the left side of her head, and for a couple of days she had some weakness of the right hand. She remained in hospital for a few weeks. On one of his visits, Foster was inspired to ask the patient to draw a face. To his astonishment, and her embarrassment, she executed a sketch such as a 4-year-old might make. Day after day she practised and gradually she regained her former artistic skill.

He had important things to say on the question of the speech-thought affiliation, quoting the case of an important statesman who sustained a stroke but who, for the following 30 minutes, was able to carry out his duties, thinking clearly about various topics, unaware of any intellectual disturbance. Only later, when he had occasion to speak, did he discover that he was aphasic.

Foster Kennedy's status as a wise and fashionable consultant, a friend and confidant of the élite, was known to me. In his chauffeur-driven, open limousine, he was an impressive figure, conspicuous with his sombrero. He became an authority not only in the realm of neurology but also in some affairs of state. Some of the invasive physical attempts at treating psychoneurotic disorders aroused his strong criticism.

Like most "pure" neurologists, Foster Kennedy was strongly opposed to Freudian ideas and treatments. He never ceased to assert that when one is mentally ill something must be wrong with the brain. He even cautiously welcomed some of the less traumatic physical efforts at the cure of patients with psychotic disorders. When in 1938 an American edition of Sagel's book on Insulin Therapy appeared, translated by Samuel Wortis, Kennedy wrote a preface, in which he said . . . "In Vienna at least one man had revolted from the obsession that only psychological remedies can ever benefit psychological ills; had refused to turn his back on modern methods to fight mental ailments, to use only the same weapons that the Greeks had used—though the Greeks used them better. The scholasticism of our time is being blown away by a new wind and whatever may be the verdict of the next decade in reference to Manfred Sagel's contribution to the treatment of so-called "schizophrenia" we shall not again be minister to a mind diseased merely by philosophy and words."

Were Foster Kennedy still living, I believe he would consider that the "new wind" had probably blown itself out.

We must have exchanged letters and reprints, for we had many interests in common. My first clear memory of meeting Foster Kennedy was in 1949, at the time of the 4th International Congress of Neurology in Paris. The following year he came to London, and on 18th July 1950 he lectured at the National Hospital. The next day he joined me on a ward round, and over coffee he chatted in a fascinating manner with the post-graduate students. A group photograph was taken in the garden of Queen Square with Foster Kennedy in the centre of a group of students. When I told him that I was planning to visit America the following year, he gave me a cordial invitation to call on him.

My next contact was both indirect and unorthodox. A close friend of mine—we had been medical students together—told me that he intended to visit New York. Accustomed to foreign travel, he had not taken kindly to post-war restrictions. At that time, that is 1950, there was still considerable austerity in England as well as stringent currency restrictions. It was virtually impossible to travel abroad merely for pleasure. Nevertheless, my friend proposed to do so and he had already bought his return ticket. When I asked how he expected to survive in the States, he assured me there would be no problem for he had good contacts there.

A week later I had a personal telephone call from New York with the charges reversed. It was my friend, who was at his wits' end. Although he had his return ticket, he was unable to pay his hotel bill. What could he do? My advice was that he should call upon Foster Kennedy, tell him I had sent him, and explain frankly his predicament. He did so, and Foster Kennedy was most sympathetic and generous. This was the beginning of a cordial amity between Foster Kennedy and my fellow student.

On his return to England, I asked my friend how he came to be in such a plight. His reply was startling and salutary. Before leaving home he had bought, at no little expense, a rare postage stamp, which he put inside his pocket diary. Arriving in New York, he went to a commercial philatelist and offered it for sale. To his dismay, he was told that the stamp was a worthless fake. He knew no one in New York, and had telephoned me for advice. Foster had most nobly come to his assistance.

On 12th April 1951 I arrived at New York, en route for an engagement as Visiting Professor to the University of California, San Francisco. I telephoned Foster Kennedy, who kindly invited me to stay for a few days at his house in Sutton Square. Of course, I was delighted. He lived in what must be one of the most desirable locations in Manhattan. The Square is in a cul de sac, the bottom of which overlooks the East River. The house was typically Georgian in style, and at the rear was a lawn with trees and flowering shrubs. It was like being in Chelsea or Clifton. The Square had become fashionable since 1921, when the daughter of J.P. Morgan came to live there.

Foster and his second wife, Katherine, greeted me warmly. He was not seeing any patients because his health had not been good. Indeed, the diagnosis of polyarteritis nodosa had recently been made. The first symptoms had appeared a year earlier, during the Neurological Congress in Paris. He had developed pain in his ankle, and palpation had brought to his notice a tender nodule lying on the epicondyle. When he returned to New York, he sought advice and the nature of his problem had been revealed.

Day after day we gossiped, recalling neurologists of the past and exchanging small talk of mutual interest. In his New York practice he seemed to have met everyone of note—politicians, writers, artists, and especially actors and actresses. Many of them became his personal friends. Winston Churchill, for example, whom he had seen after he had been knocked down by a car, came under his care and later dined with him at Sutton Square.

We talked about his house. When he had bought the property in 1919, the area was run-down and dilapidated; a rubbish dump lay where there was now a lawn.

Foster asked about my plans. I intended to reach San Francisco by a roundabout route, stopping off at Virginia Beach to attend the annual meeting of the International League Against Epilepsy. At the time I was President of the British branch. Then I would make my way to Mexico City, staying en route at New Orleans and Miami Beach. Foster gave me letters of introduction to Dr. Mareno and to Dr. Orapeso, both of whom lived in Mexico City. He asked if I was likely to visit Los Angeles, and when I said I might attend a symposium there, he gave me a letter to Edmund Gwenn, the British film actor. Mr. Gwenn did indeed call for me and took me to dine in a Hollywood restaurant.

My plan was to return from San Francisco by train to Chicago, and then fly to New York. Foster asked me to stay with him again for a few days before leaving for London. When I was in California, I heard from time to time the worrying news that he was not at all well. On landing at Idlewild, I was handed a message to the effect that Foster was in hospital but that he had arranged for me to stay as his guest at the River Club, close to Sutton Square.

Straightway I went to see him in the Doctors' Hospital. He was in a poor state, but seemed bright and cheerful and eager to talk. He told me that some weeks previously he had woken in the night feeling that something had "gone wrong". Then he realised that he could scarcely move one arm and one leg, those limbs feeling heavy. His speech was unaffected, and he could grimace and move his tongue normally. He realised, too, that there was also something the matter with his "normal" arm and leg. After switching on the bedside light he got hold of his tiepin, which was on the table beside the bed. On testing himself he discovered that the pinpricks felt blunt over his "normal" limbs and the corresponding half of his trunk, but were quite sharp over the paretic limbs. "I realised", he told me, "that I had developed a Brown-Séquard syndrome, presumably due to a nodule in the cervical region of my spinal cord."

By the time I saw him the neurological signs had lessened somewhat, and he invited me to lunch with him at the hospital the next day. This was 15th June 1951.

Foster improved to the extent that he was allowed to return to Sutton Square. An electric chair-lift had been installed and attached to the balustrade.

I stayed on at the River Club, but dined each evening at Sutton Square. For much of the time Foster rested in his bedroom, but at about 6 o'clock he would come downstairs in his dressing gown. Seated in his armchair with a trolley in front of him, he performed a slow and solemn ritual of preparing cocktails for the three of us.

Although frail, Foster remained a splendid host. He was witty in discourse and our conversation touched upon cabbages and Kings. We must surely have discussed Oscar Wilde, one of my literary obsessions. A short but critical biography had appeared in 1951 by an old friend of his, St.John Ervine, who had dedicated the book to Foster and Katherine.

The monarchs of neurology were one of our favourite topics. Although I was Gowers's biographer, I had never met that great man. Foster, however, had worked with him, and coped with all his foibles at first hand. All this was absorbing information.

Foster strongly disapproved of psycho-analysis. In wartime France he had encountered many cases of battle neurosis, and had written much upon its nature and treatment. I believe that Foster favoured and even practised electro-convulsive therapy in patients with depression but he never discussed the matter with me.

We shared certain anxieties about the practice of spinal anaesthesia, for we both had experience of serious and permanent complications in patients following such procedures.

There appeared at that time to be no method of avoiding such grave after-effects. Both of us had written papers on the subject.

In February 1952 his illness worsened, and an abrupt intestinal haemorrhage necessitated his admission to the Bellevue Hospital. In the ward where he had for so long laboured and taught, he died on 7th February 1952, a few days before his 68th birthday.

Foster Kennedy was one of the finest British ambassadors to the United States. He came, he saw, he conquered; unlike Julius Caesar, he remained in the country of his adoption, a loved and highly honoured citizen.

Perhaps it is not inappropriate to quote what "The New York Times" had to say:

> One of the leading personalities of the United States and the world for many years, Dr. Kennedy was more than an outstanding physician or neurologist. He was a scholar and a wit, connoisseur and philosopher, an accomplished orator and raconteur. The mere announcement that Foster Kennedy was to deliver an address or participate in a discussion was sufficient to assure a lecture-hall over-crowded by fellow-physicians, whom he never failed to delight with his original point of view, his fresh approach to a problem, his *bons mots* and aphorisms, pronounced in a faint Irish brogue. The medical fraternity came to regard him as a modern version of a Delphic oracle who always could be counted upon to highlight the essence of a subject with a trenchant quotable phrase.

1879–1955
René Leriche

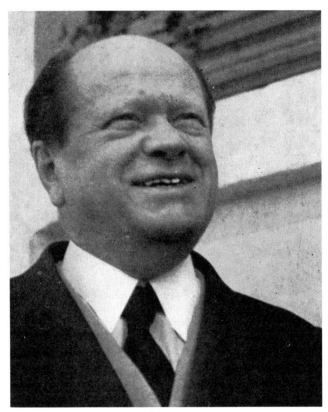

RENÉ LERICHE

From Leriche, R: *Souvenirs de ma Vie Morte*. Editions du Seuil, Paris, 1956.

In 1934 my medical school honoured me with an invitation to deliver the Long Fox Lecture. The choice of subject was important. It should be neurological, but yet appeal widely. The many obscure aspects of that universal experience—pain—immediately suggested itself, and that was the topic I chose.

What was the purpose of pain, if any? Some ecclesiastics were still nursing the opinion that pain is a punishment, as its etymology suggests. But why should dumb animals be afflicted by intolerable agony through faults not of their own? Pain as a sentinel indicating the presence of some putative danger that calls for action, is too facile. What of *tic douloureux* where the spasms of intense suffering are meaningless? What are the mental and bodily effects of severe and prolonged pain? Are they specific or not? And does pain-endurance bring about a kind of spiritual cleansing, as some theists and even a few doctors have claimed?

Of all the theorists who had written about this important theme, Leriche seemed to me to stand alone. One of his statements was: "To every individual and his entourage, an illness is a disaster. Even the most straightforward surgical intervention entails a brutal assault upon delicate connective tissues and sensitive living structures complete with vasomotor components."

These were the words of a perceptive and humane doctor. Leriche went further. He declared that the malaise that follows even the simplest surgical measure often endures for many months. There is, he said, "a post-operative malady" or syndrome resulting from tissue-trauma. This disability is neither inevitable nor unavoidable. It can be minimized, if not circumvented, by operative techniques that are unhurried, deliberate, meticulously careful, with minimal bruising and blood-loss.

Such was the compassionate philosopher whom the world was acclaiming in 1934 as the "pain-surgeon" par excellence.

Many of Leriche's papers upon this topic were known to me and eagerly studied. It was not until 1940 that his classic monograph *La Chirurgerie de la Douleur* was published by Masson of Paris. According to Leriche, "Physical pain is no simple affair of an impulse travelling at a fixed rate along a nerve. It is the resultant of a conflict between a stimulus and the whole individual. The problem of pain represents a "conglomeration of obscurities"."

In another place and at another time, he had likened operating surgeons to taxi-drivers. The fastest are not the best, but rather those who choose the least busy route, who avoid obstacles and who get you safely to your destination.

Leriche's views about pain, though applauded, did not receive the recognition they deserved. Today they are largely forgotten. The advent of more "scientific" ideas about the pathophysiology of pain-mechanisms has overshadowed many of Leriche's philosophic attitudes. In particular, the notion of a chemistry of pain is attracting most attention.

Leriche believed that the autonomic nervous system plays an important role in the production and transmission of pain. He devoted much attention to disorders of the vascular system and to the possibility of their relief by surgical intervention directed at various levels of the sympathetic system.

Who was this unconventional thinker and innovator? At the time I was preparing my lecture, he had been, since 1924, occupying the Chair of Surgery at Strasbourg (but in 1931 he returned to his medical school in Lyons as Professor of Surgery). In 1936 he attained the highest possible post, namely that of Professor of the Collège de France in Paris. This exalted office, established about 1530 by Francis I, had been held by such notables as Claude-Bernard, Brown-Séquard and Henri Bergson. Leriche was in office for 15 years. His inaugural address was on "The Surgery of Pain". Other honours were accorded him. He became a member of the Académie des Sciences, and, a week later, of the Académie Nationale de Médecine. He was by then a Grand Officer of the Légion d'Honneur, and the President of the Société de Biologie; he was also the recipient of many honorary doctorates and medals.

Up to now I had never met Leriche in person. I had not visited the University of Lyons and our paths had not crossed, although I knew quite well the attractive city of Strasbourg. Leriche's former colleague, the dignified and distinguished Professor J.A. Barré, was a good friend of mine. Leriche's successor, Professor Weiss—surely one of the most elegant and cultured figures in French medicine—I knew well.

When I became Dean of the Institute of Neurology in 1948, I established the practice of inviting guest lecturers to the National Hospital, Queen Square. The honorarium was small, but no one refused an invitation.

On 4th July 1949, Professor Leriche lectured at my request. The following day we had lunch at the Royal Society of Medicine, and in the evening I arranged a dinner party in his honour at the Connaught Hotel. The other guests were Sir Francis Walshe, Harold Edwards (surgeon to Kings' College Hospital), Sir Heneage Ogilvie (surgeon to Guy's Hospital), Julian Taylor (neurosurgeon, University College Hospital) and Fergus Ferguson (neurologist to Manchester Royal Infirmary).

Leriche was a most attractive man of somewhat unusual appearance. He was short, stocky and clean-shaven. The top of his head was bald with a crescent of untidy hair, giving a halo-like appearance. With his ready smile and his rather bulbous nose he could, with no disrespect, be likened to a comedian. His English was fluent, and his conversation entertaining. His lecture in London was highly successful and he was a most congenial companion.

Our next meeting was in Paris in November 1950, when he invited me to lunch with him at his apartment. I believe he was living in rue d'Alboni, near the Trocadero and close by the

Pont Bir-Hakeim. On entering his study, I noticed with interest a painting, obviously by Vlaminck, of a floral arrangement. I, too, had a flower piece by Vlaminck in my consulting rooms in London. The flowers were different in the two paintings, but the pewter jug which held the flowers was identical. I remarked upon this to Leriche, who said, "But have you seen my Matisse?" He opened a drawer and took out a magnificent sketch of his own head. "Matisse came to see me the other day", Leriche said, "and asked why I had not framed the picture and displayed it on the wall. I told him that my wife thought the picture was nothing like me. 'Maybe not', said Matisse, 'but it's like you will be.' "

Leriche died towards the end of 1955, and, to my regret, I had not seen him again. A few years later I was in San Francisco and visited an exhibition of Matisse's work. On the wall hung the picture of Leriche.

It was not until later that I learned some details of his life. In the first place, I read his autobiography, *Souvenirs de ma vie morte,* published posthumously in 1956 by the Editions du Seuil, Paris. The other source was M. Maurice Chevassu, who delivered the eloquent éloge before the Académie Nationale de Médecine.

René Leriche was born at Roanne (Loire) on 12th October 1879. There were many doctors on both the paternal and maternal sides of his family. Like Alajouanine, he was educated by the Marist Fathers, first at Roanne and later at Saint-Chamond. When he was a child, an uncle, interested in phrenology, felt his bumps and proclaimed that he should be a surgeon. At an early age, René had more romantic aspirations and wanted to enter Saint-Cyr, become an Army officer, and explore Africa. His ideas changed when he was a little older and he became more attuned to philosophy. He spent a year's retreat within la Trappe-de-sept-Fons, a step he never regretted. He then entered the Faculty of Science at the University of Lyons, transferring to the medical school a year later.

This period coincided with his term of military service, part of which he spent as extern to Professor Poncet, a well-known surgeon in Lyons.

It was at this time he began his friendship with Alexis Carrel, a doctor six years his senior. This famous man had already started his research work on suturing arteries, before leaving Lyons for New York. In due course he became a Nobel laureate. The last ten years of Carrel's life were spent in France where—rightly or wrongly—he was regarded as a collaborator with the German occupying force.

At the end of his military service, Leriche became an intern; after that, for six years, a *chef de clinique* to the skilful Professor Délore, ". . . one of the best surgeons I ever knew".

Leriche was now a close friend of Paul Cavaillon ". . . not a very dextrous technician, but what a brain!". The two of them began to spend working holidays together abroad, visiting Swiss and German clinics. They came to realise the inadequacies of the medical facilities in Lyons. By resorting to anonymous letters to the Press, they tried to rectify some of the defects. It must have been at this period that Leriche met Emil Kocher of Berne, the gentleness of whose technique was so impressive. In 1909 Kocher also became a Nobel Prize winner.

French doctors were reputed to be reluctant to journey abroad, but Leriche was an outstanding exception. From the age of 17 he travelled throughout the world and became one of the most attractive emissaries of French thinking.

An early visit to the United States brought him in touch with the surgeon who probably exercised the greatest influence upon his professional life. As Oscar Wilde said, "In Art, as in everything, *on est toujours le fils de quel qu'un*". This father-figure was William Halsted, who, since 1889, had been Chief of Surgery at Johns Hopkins Hospital, Baltimore. Halsted was probably the first, and certainly the supreme, exponent of delicate, slow, bloodless technique in surgery. His influence on Leriche, coupled with that exercised earlier by Kocher and later by Cushing, was life-long. Apart from these professional influences, Leriche learned his exquisite skill with sutures from the old women lace-makers in the villages around Lyons.

With the onset of the 1914 war, Leriche was put in charge of surgery at the Hôpital du Carlton, organised by the White Russian colony in Paris under the direction of General Poliakoff and his wife. In 1917, however, he was seconded to a special unit at Bouleuse, near Rheims. This was to be a centre for the intensive study of war wounds, and for the instruction of medical officers in the latest advances in treatment. Many famous specialists were on the staff, including Georges Guillain, the future Charcot Professor of Neurology.

With the Armistice, Leriche returned to Lyons. At this point he was offered the Chair of Surgery at Strasbourg, which was once again a French city. Leriche declined, but six years later it was offered to him a second time. On this occasion he accepted, and hc and his wife established themselves in the Maison Voltaire—where, incidentally, pâté de fois gras en croûte had first been prepared. Strasbourg, it may be said, is one of the most attractive cities in Europe. Its medical facilities are housed within a quaint old *cité hospitalaire,* with its flowers and trees forming a great garden. Like Lyons, Strasbourg is renowned for its cuisine and wines. Leriche was indeed fortunate.

There he collaborated with Jung upon the subject of phlebitis, and with Fontaine upon the practice of sympathectomy for the relief of pain. His researches into arteriovenous surgery led clinicians to recognise a "syndrome de Leriche", which entails a partial or total occlusion of the abdominal aorta at the point of its bifurcation.

In 1928 Foerster and Wilder Penfield visited Leriche. Each morning for three days they watched him operate, and each evening they dined with him and his wife. They admired his dexterity, and they listened to his fascinating peroration while he was scrubbing his hands before the operation on the first morning. On the second day, to their astonishment, he repeated his talk with unabated eloquence, as South American surgeons came crowding in to watch him. And on the third day, word for word, he made the same speech. The following day, Penfield and Foerster lunched alone. Mellowed by the surroundings and by the wine, Foerster "reproduced Leriche's introductory speech, word for word, in perfect French, complete with gestures, and we laughed and laughed . . .".

In 1936 came Leriche's election to the Collège de France. It was required of him to deliver 20 addresses over a ten-year period. Leriche decided upon a programme, starting with pain, proceeding thence to researches on bony tissue (the product of his wartime studies at Bouleuse), and thence to lesions of arteries and veins. His concluding lecture dealt with "The Philosophy of Surgery", which appeared as a monograph published by Flammarion.

One further publication epitomized Leriche's surgical thought, *The Fundamentals of Physiological Surgery* (Masson, 1955). Owing to a long-standing dispute between the Collège de France and the University of Paris, there were no facilities for him to carry out clinical work locally. With increasing difficulty, therefore, he commuted between Strasbourg and Paris, a state of affairs which continued until the outbreak of the Second World War in 1939. The University of Strasbourg was then evacuated to Clérmond-Ferrand, and Professor and Mme. Leriche took the last train out of the city, leaving behind them the Maison Voltaire—which they hoped would remain intact until the war ended.

Now aged 60, Leriche was asked what he would like to do and he requested a centre for vascular surgery to be set up in the Maginot Line. The site was not approved and was located within the Hôpital Grange-Blanche in Lyons.

With the collapse of France, Leriche's difficulties must have started. He was already well-known to Marshal Pétain because in 1934 he had seen Marshal Joffre, Pétain's close friend, who was suffering from arteritis in one leg. After gangrene set in, a mid-thigh amputation became necessary but Marshal Joffre had died shortly afterwards. In 1940 Pétain took the terrible decision to capitulate to Hitler. He then became Chief of State with dictatorial powers over that part of France which remained unoccupied. Leriche, therefore, was subjected to Pétain's authority. Reluctant to conform, Leriche refused the post of Minister of Health, and also that of Education. Then came a threat that French doctors might be deported to Germany. Leriche therefore accepted the important post of Director of Medical Services, and, on Pétain's instructions, moved from Lyons to Paris.

There he was granted facilities to continue surgical work at the well-run American Hospital, under the direction of Général de Chambrun. He worked there until the end of the war. Three times a week he attended the Collège de France.

Although it is nowhere emphasized, Leriche must have been in an invidious position with regard to the Army of Occupation and the Resistance. The Vichy authorities offered him a Chair at the Salpêtrière, which he refused. He also rejected the offer of a surgical service at the Hôpital Necker. Leriche moreover refused promotion to the rank of Commander of the Légion d'Honneur.

After the war, with advancing years Leriche became increasingly sensitive to the cold, and he regularly spent the winter months in his Mediterranean villa at Cassis. On Christmas Day 1955 he received shattering news. A telephone call from Marseilles informed him that his old crony, Fiolle, had suddenly died. In great distress, he raced across to the stricken home to bring comfort to the bereaved daughters. The emotional strain was too much, and on 29th December René Leriche succumbed to a massive heart attack.

He was buried in the cemetry of Saint-Foy-les-Lyon, adjoining the hill of Fourvière, not far from his birthplace. His had, indeed, been a full life and a happy one, and he received the recognition that was due to him. He was a most exceptional man. It is to be hoped that his real greatness will not be forgotten in this present era of scientific endeavour.

If anything I have written will revive and perpetuate the acclaim due to Leriche, the philosopher-surgeon of pain, I shall be content.

1877–1959
Jean Lhermitte

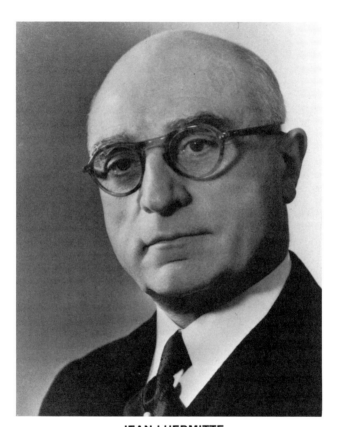

JEAN LHERMITTE

From Critchley, M: *Parietal Lobes*. Edward Arnold, London, 1953.

The name and work of Professor Jean Lhermitte first became familiar to me in the Spring of 1923, when I joined Maida Vale Hospital for Epilepsy and Paralysis as its Resident Medical Officer. Two Registrars were appointed at the same time, Philip Cloake and Douglas McAlpine. The latter had just finished a six-month period in Paris, studying the pathology of post-encephalitic Parkinsonism. There he had been under the immediate supervision of Professor Lhermitte, of whose abilities and personality he was enthusiastic. While I was still at Maida Vale, I became friendly with George Riddoch, one of the consultant physicians. He too knew Lhermitte; indeed, they were close friends. I am eternally grateful to Riddoch for his letter of introduction to Professor Lhermitte on my behalf a few years later.

My opportunity to meet him came in 1928, after my lecture at the Préfecture de Police. I called on him in his apartment in the rue Marboeuf, where, across the street, resided the venerable André-Thomas.

Lhermitte greeted me with considerable warmth. His appearance was striking. He was a rather short man, clean-shaven and bald-headed. Indeed, such few hairs that remained were so close-cropped as to be inconspicuous. He had a largish nose and mouth, and as he talked his features lit up with animation. In repose, a violent tic-like spasm would now and then dart across his face. He talked with vivacity and exuberance, and his gestures were somewhat extravagant.

Despite his loquacity, he was an attentive listener. Unlike the syndrome of "brainy verbosity", which I have described as a feature of such men as Lord Macaulay, he did not monopolise the interview. He was a stimulating conversationalist; what he had to say was full of wisdom, and, to my relief, couched in fluent English.

How old was Lhermitte when I first met him? I could not guess, for, with his almost total lack of hair, he seemed ageless. What I can affirm is that, over the ensuing period of more than 30 years when I was meeting him frequently, he did not seem to grow older either physically or mentally.

It did not take me long to realise that Lhermitte was an exceptional man. His range of knowledge was immense, and his enthusiasm was contagious. As a polymath with a flair for the new, the unusual and the unexpected, he was a veritable Dr. Casaubon. If there was ever such an entity as neuropsychiatry, Jean Lhermitte was its High Priest. He had studied and mastered every part of it from the foundations and basements to the roof-tops.

His earliest researches had been morphological and anatomo-pathological. From clinical neurology, his interests had widened and became increasingly psycho-pathological. He eagerly studied that ill-defined frontier between medicine and religion. In the territory of mental activity, nothing was too obscure or too *caché* for him to neglect. And with all these multitudinous interests there was the fervour and gusto which over-flowed into his abundant zeal to communicate. In so doing he showed no tendency to tyrannize, domineer or eclipse, like so many garrulous pundits.

It was Lhermitte's interest in the neurological syndromes of the aged which first appealed to me. When in 1930 I was preparing my Goulstonian Lectures upon the neurology of old age, it was to Paris that I once again turned to visit Lhermitte.

He asked me to join him on his hospital rounds. I called for him early at his apartment, and he summoned his regular taxi. Apparently he had no car. We made a slight detour in order to pick up Mlle. Gabrielle Lévy. Her name was familiar to me because of her work on post-encephalitis. Mlle. Lévy was crippled with multiple sclerosis, and walked only with difficulty.

Professor Lhermitte was most caring, and he arranged transport for her to and from the hospital. Later, the taxi also collected Dr. de Massary, who was one of the assistants at the hospital.

Our destination was the Hospice Paul Brousse, located in the suburb of Villejuif, beyond the Porte d'Italie. The patients within the hospice comprised the chronic sick—mainly victims of some neurological disorder—and the very aged.

Working among this grim company of disabled and decaying humanity, was the intern, a young lady of outstanding beauty. Lhermitte was obviously worried about one of his patients who was desperately ill. He quietly took aside the glamorous lady doctor and asked how the patient was getting on. The intern made no reply but shrugged her shoulders and emitted a "raspberry"-like noise. Lhermitte did not react, but I was disillusioned.

Some of the sad and even grotesque victims I can still vividly recall. There was a man who appeared to have a Victoria plum half inside and half outside his mouth. He was a ticqueur who had been afflicted by spells of involuntary protrusion of the tongue. In an effort to control this lingual tic, he had closed his lips so tightly upon the extruded tongue that strangulation resulted. The tip swelled to such a degree that it could not be drawn back into the mouth. Speech was impossible; so was mastication, and he had to be kept alive by intranasal feeds.

The Hospice Paul Brousse apparently existed outside the University dominion, and Lhermitte worked there as Médecin-Chef in relative isolation. He was, however, in charge of the Dejerine Laboratory for Brain Research at the Salpêtrière, where postgraduate students came from all parts of the world to work with him.

Early in his career he had published an important monograph on *La Paraplégie des Vieillards*. At the turn of the century in Allbut & Rollerston's *System of Medicine,* there had appeared a brief article on "Senile Paraplegia", as though there existed a clear-cut syndrome. Lhermitte used no such term, but referred to weakness of the legs *in old people.* He argued that difficulty in walking might result from senescent changes at various levels of the neuraxis, cortical, basal, cerebellar, spinal, neuritic, and even in the muscles themselves. Indeed, in any one patient there might co-exist lesions occurring simultaneously at several different sites. This idea tallied exactly with my experience as the result of examining a large number of nonagenarians and some centenarians.

Gradually, as our friendship grew, I came to learn something of Jean Lhermitte's background. Like so many neurologists working at that time in Paris, he had been born outside the metropolis. His birthplace was Mont-Saint-Père (Aisne). His father had been a professional artist, a member of the Barbizon school of landscape painters whose number included Rousseau, Daubigny, Diaz de la Peña, and—more remotely—Corot and Millet. Jean Lhermitte himself did not paint, as far as I know, but he understood something of the anatomy of art. One of his early publications was *L'oeil du Peintre* (The Painter's Eye).

As a young medical man, Lhermitte had been closely associated with Henri Claude, the Professor of Psychiatry in Paris. During his time "under the shadow of the dome of the Salpêtrière", as Alajouanine put it, Lhermitte did much original work in neuropathology. He perfected a method for staining microscopic preparations. With Gustave Roussy, he wrote an important monograph upon "Anatomo-pathological techniques". While still at this stage in his career, he published papers upon the subject of trans-section of the spinal cord. The so-called Lhermitte's sign—also known as the barber's chair phenomenon—has proved to be a valuable diagnostic adjunct to the neurologist, being highly suggestive of multiple sclerosis.

His interests became progressively more penetrating. Many of the unusual phenomena associated with sleep began to fascinate him. Narcolepsy, cataplexy, predormital hallucinations, sleep- and waking-paralysis, all these came under his scrutiny. Symptoms stemming from mesencephalic disorders began to intrigue him. He was the first to describe the phenomenon of Lilliputian hallucinations associated with lesions within the interpeduncular space.

Then his interest turned to the body-image, culminating in the appearance of his fascinating book *L'Image de notre Corps*. This preoccupation led him into reflections upon phantom limbs, asomatognosia, disordered spatial conceptions and geometric apractagnosia. Of special note was his consideration of such unusual events as specular hallucinoses, which he spoke of as autoscopy or heautoscopy.

Once again, his father's profession asserted itself in his thinking, and one of his later papers was entitled: "New psychophysiological considerations upon painting: the body-image in pictorial space".

Over the many years in which I knew Lhermitte and talked to him, I was amazed by the breadth of his interests and the profundity of his knowledge. There was only one aspect of neurology in which, apparently, he was not engrossed, and that was aphasia. Yet his brilliant son, François, is today one of the world's most outstanding aphasiologists.

Professor Jean Lhermitte had had a religious upbringing, and in his maturity he was fascinated by many topics which occupy the hinterland between mind and soul. He was in the habit each year of attending a study group where such themes were considered in detail. The proceedings were published in a series of monographs known as *Les Etudes Carmelitiennes*. One year, demoniacal possession came under close investigation, and the outcome was the monograph *Satan*. Another year, stigmatization was discussed. The historical development of ideas concerning a supposed seat of the emotions was thoroughly explored in the Etude entitled *Le Coeur*.

Naturally, Lhermitte and I lost touch with each other during the 1939–1946 war, but, as soon as Paris was retaken by de Gaulle's forces and the American army, I wrote to him. He replied telling me that he had carried on his neuropsychiatric duties under great difficulties. He had worked as Consultant-Intern at the Hospice Paul Brousse. Presumably, he meant he lived in at the hospital. A few months later, while I was still in the Royal Navy, I visited him in Paris along with my psychiatric colleague Surgeon Captain Desmond Curran. There were distressing shortages of food and comforts, and I enquired whether I could send him anything from England. His one request was for a copy of Hugh Trevor-Roper's *The Last Days of Hitler.*

In 1947 came his recognition from the University of Paris, when he was accorded the rank of honorary Professor.

He resumed his busy private practice in the rue Marboeuf. He had also acquired a country home at Arcachon, near the Spanish border, on the French Basque coastline.

For many years, invitations had come from London requesting him to lecture. In November 1934 he stayed with George Riddoch and lectured at the National Hospital on the subject of spino-cerebellar degeneration. He also addressed the student Listerian Society at Kings' College Hospital, taking as his theme the life and work of Charcot. The six of us who comprised the Hexagon Club invited him to dine and afterwards to chat informally on a variety of neurological matters, but, in particular, on spinal concussion.

Year after year I continued to visit Professor Lhermitte. He was so warm-hearted and friendly. At the same time,· I found his conversation to be so stimulating. Out-of-the-way subjects, off-beat and arcane, have always appealed to me, and here I found a like-minded thinker, as evidenced by his exuberant comments and observations. As far as I can remember, we rarely visited restaurants. Usually I dined with him *en famille,* in the company of his most gracious wife and often his son and daughter. The only other "outsider" I can recall joining us was his brilliant protegé of Basque origin, Dr. de Ajuriaguerra.

Elsewhere I have described Lhermitte as the most learned and versatile expert in Europe on diseases of the nervous system. He was the veritable Sage of neurology. Eloquent, excitable, vivacious, infectious with his perpetual ebullience, he was a man of tremendous learning who brought deep philosophical thinking to almost all aspects of neurology.

His hospitality was extended to my elder son, then a student at the Sorbonne, who had the enjoyable experience of staying with him at Arcachon.

Lhermitte continued in active practice and at literary work well into old age. His final years were handicapped by a visual disorder. He died, quietly, in his sleep, on 24th January 1959.

Walter Riese, that erudite man of Richmond, Virginia, wrote of his old chief, Professor Lhermitte: "Rarely, if ever, did the history of neurology produce a figure reflecting with equal force the continuity and unity of life, man, and work."

1902–1977
Alexander Romanovich Luria

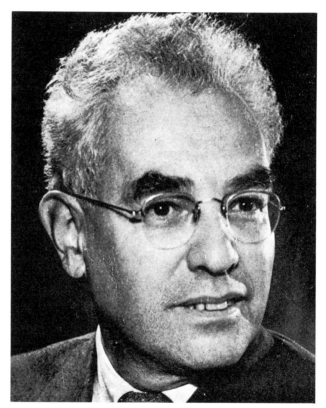

ALEXANDER ROMANOVICH LURIA

From Critchley, M: *Aphasiology.* Edward Arnold, London, 1970.

On 2nd August 1931, I disembarked from a paddle-steamer on the Volga river at the industrial city of Kazan, capital of the Tatar autonomous republic of the U.S.S.R. I knew that the University boasted of such students as Tolstoy and Lenin, the latter having been sent down for misbehaviour, but I did not know then that it was the birthplace of my future friend, Alexander Romanovich Luria. Indeed, at that time I had not heard of him. The weather was scorchingly hot and our stop-over was no longer than one hour. I was glad to return to the comparative cool of the boat en route for Samara and Stalingrad.

My first dealings with Luria were in 1960, and by post. I had been given the task of organising a formal discussion upon "Aphasia", to take place at the 7th International Congress of Neurology in Rome in 1961. It was necessary for me to select the principal speakers. Luria was among those I invited, and he accepted immediately.

For some years I had been aware of his refreshing and thoughtful papers upon this subject. I found him to be, like me, a half-hearted localizationist; nevertheless, he did venture a partial classification of the aphasias. His frequent reference to Pavlov and Pavlovian ideas was slightly irritating, even though it was less marked than in most other Russian writers. Luria had worked with L.E. Vygotsky, whose monograph *Thought and Language* I possessed and admired.

It transpired that Luria was unable to attend the conference in person, but he sent me the typescript of his address and it was read for him. His paper aroused considerable interest, and neurologists eagerly awaited further papers from him.

135

In 1963 the Ciba Foundation in London organised a three-day symposium upon disorders of language, and asked me to preside. The speakers included neurologists such as Russell Brain and Henri Hécaen; the linguist Roman Jakobson and the philosopher Suzanne Langer. Psychology was represented by Professor Oliver Zangwill. Luria also agreed to participate, but unfortunately once again he was prevented from attending. He sent me his manuscript, which I read on his behalf.

Later that same year, on 22nd November, Luria came to England. He visited the National Hospital, and accompanied me on a teaching ward-round. Next day he was a guest lecturer at the hospital, and I was privileged to preside. The following evening I arranged a small dinner-party in his honour at the Garrick Club. Francis Walshe, Russell Brain and Oliver Zangwill were my other guests. On 25th November I delivered the Victor Horsley Lecture on "The Problem of Visual Agnosia", and Luria was present. It was at this point that he invited me to visit his clinic in Moscow and to stay for at least a month.

I had spent some time in Moscow in 1931 and had no desire to revisit that city. At the time I had wanted to see Lenin's widow, Krupskaya, but, although I had a personal letter of introduction to her, no one seemed to know where she was. However, on taking up Professor Luria's invitation, any unpleasant memories of 30 years earlier were completely eradicated.

Except as an aphasiologist, Luria was not well-known to me then. Gradually, however, I learned that he had attained his great prestige in neuro-psychology by a circuitous route. Sociology was his first love. There was then a brief affair with psychoanalysis. Then came short contact with Pavlovian philosophy, and with the reflexology of Bechterew. Child development intrigued him for years, together with researches into cultural anthropology in Soviet Asia. A long spell working with mental defectives followed. By the time the U.S.S.R. entered the war in 1942, Luria had also become medically qualified and he was sent to a centre for head injuries in the Urals. This was the beginning of his study of the effects of localized injuries of the brain.

This was the man who greeted me at Moscow airport on 8th June 1964.

He was of above medium height, grey-haired and clean-shaven, with an engaging, friendly expression. His upper incisor teeth were somewhat prominent, and his appearance was that of a benevolent and brainy rabbit. I soon found him to be a warm, boyish individual with a keen sense of humour. He emitted an atmosphere of friendliness and kindliness. Behind this was a stupendous intellect, and a creativity that was also enthusiastically receptive to unexplored ideas.

His spoken English was fluent—he told me he was self-taught—but naturally he had greater difficulties with the written language. He was extremely generous and hospitable to me. I was a frequent visitor to his apartment, which was situated in the centre of Moscow not far from Red Square. It was small and cluttered with furniture, and there was a bed in every room. He was fortunate in that he owned a car and had a driver. Furthermore, he owned a *dacha*, or country cottage, outside Moscow near a lake. I never saw his *dacha*, but for our dinner-parties in Moscow he would often produce some delicious lake-fish, which was probably burbot.

He shared his apartment with his wife, who was medically qualified and who was engaged on cancer-research, and with his daughter and her husband. There was a great deal of photographic equipment in the rooms.

I was accommodated in the fairly new Minsk Hotel in Gorki Street. My bedroom was bright and pleasant. Breakfast was the only meal I had there—or tried to have, for much patience and even ingenuity was required before one was served. The restaurant contained many small, round tables, on each one of which was a flag. Usually I seated myself at a table with the Union flag and then awaited events. After at least thirty minutes I might be served with tea and a hard-boiled egg. Thinking I might accelerate service if I adopted a different nationality, I sat next day at a table displaying the flag of China. That was no better. Subsequently, I utilized the flags of Poland, Hungary and even Cuba. The service did not improve, so I resumed my proper nationality.

The Bourdenko Institute, where Luria worked, was within easy walking distance. It was a neurosurgical hospital comprising some 360 beds, and Luria was in charge of the Section of Psychology.

His department was not large. When I worked there he had only two assistants, both of them women. The senior was a cheerful, motherly lady named Homskaya; the other, Vinarskaya, was younger.

As I wrote on a later occasion: "Luria's researches were carried out in an office which was more like a busy air terminal than the sanctum of a reflective scholar. Doors to the right and to the left of him opened and shut. Bells rang. All and sundry—nurses, technicians, porters, assistants—seemed to use his study like a public highway. Privacy there was none. Luria's careful case-studies were impervious to noise and distraction."

Deaf and blind to the surrounding chaos, Luria worked on like one possessed, totally oblivious to the passage of time. Sometimes he visited the wards; but the patient under scrutiny would usually be brought to him in his very public office.

Luria was tireless, maintaining his concentration and his exuberance hour after hour. He did not require relays of tea or coffee to keep him vigilant. As midday approached, I would begin to flag. By one o'clock my blood sugar was in my boots. An hour later, Luria might show signs of halting. He would look at his watch and express surprise at the lateness of the hour. "We must go", he would say. But after the patient had been dismissed, he was often button-holed by a nursing sister or by one of his assistants. He might be asked to look at a document, or to sign a paper. Leaving his office and en route to the front hall, he might espy a patient sitting there. It would be impossible for him to pass without stopping, chatting, even perhaps carrying out a minor test-procedure.

Eventually, we escaped from the Institute and embarked upon our search for sustenance. We visited different eating places on different days. The Baku Restaurant seemed to be Luria's first choice, while I preferred the Peking Restaurant where I could always be sure of chicken à la Kiev being on the menu. Apart from caviare and borscht, this was my favourite Russian dish. Luria never drank vodka, but a glass was always awaiting me before the meal.

The method of examination Luria practised was of the pencil-and-paper type, preceded or accompanied by a searching history-taking. He carried out but little in the way of physical examination, and scarcely ever did he resort to mechanical or electrical gadgetry. Luria did not make use of the "token" test of Vignolo and de Renzi, so popular among Western European aphasiologists. His tests were, I found, ingenious and highly original.

One item of technique struck me as strange. On testing an aphasiac's ability to put a name to objects or ideas, Luria used pictorial models. He had a scrapbook with coloured pictures stuck in, and the patient was directed to name each one. In England we prefer to confront the patient with an actual test-object, allowing him to touch it, handle it or explore its shape and consistency before giving it a name. Subsequently, I decided to use both methods of testing.

These manoeuvres and the actions of the patient were recorded by me in the barrister's notebook with "legal size" paper which I had brought with me. In a few days it was filled, and I looked for a fresh supply of writing paper. None was available either in the Institute or in my hotel. I searched vainly for a stationer's shop, and then I thought of Gumm, the huge store. There I found a plethora of boots and shoes, but paper was scarce. Eventually I succeeded in buying an expensive notebook of shoddy paper.

Forty years earlier, Luria had had similar difficulties in securing paper for his journal entitled: *Problems of the Psycho-*

physiology of Labour. Finally, he obtained packages of yellow wrapping paper from a soap factory.

One of the patients we studied in detail day after day was an educated man who had been flown in from the southern part of the U.S.S.R. He had a small but invasive brain tumour located at the tip of the left frontal lobe. As the neoplasm increased, the suspicion grew that a subtle affection of speech was taking place. The idea was confirmed, the patient passing through the phase of what I called "pre-aphasia" before sustaining an obvious speech-impairment. This case was the basis for my later studies on ingravescent or impending loss of speech.

While I was working at the Bourdenko Institute, I was introduced to Professor Bein, an aphasiologist well-known to me by repute. She kindly invited me to lecture to her students, which I did, with Luria acting as interpreter.

During my stay I also met briefly the neurologist Professor Schmidt, Academician Sarkisov who had worked in the National Hospital, and Professor Tonkonogy of the Bechterew Institute in Leningrad. Luria always referred gleefully to the last-named as "Daddy Long-legs". My old friends Professor Kroll and the neuroanatomist Hindze, were never mentioned, and I tactfully did not enquire about them.

One product of my Moscow interlude was a paper written in conjunction with Luria, E.D. Homskaya and S.M. Blinkov, entitled: "Impaired Selectivity of Mental Processes in Association with a Lesion of the Frontal Lobe" and published in *Neuropsychologia,* 1967, vol. 5.

Luria made sure that my spare time was agreeably occupied. To my great delight, he took me to the ballet—at the Kremlin Congressional Hall, at the Bolshoi Theatre and at a small "musical" theatre. I watched "The Sleeping Beauty", "Giselle" (twice), "The Snow Queen", "Raymonda", and a ballet little known outside Russia, "The Stone Flower". On these occasions the audience was critical but ebullient, shouting out the name of their favourite ballerina, and, after the final curtain, running down the aisles to stand before the orchestra pit in adulation. I was taken to a concert to hear Rudolph Kerer, and we also went to the cinema to see a Russian version of "Hamlet", with Smokherovski in the title role.

Luria and I lunched at the British Embassy with our Ambassador, Sir Humphrey Trevelyan (later Lord Trevelyan). We took boat trips on the Moscow river. Once or twice we went for picnics, the most memorable being a visit to Tolstoy's country house at Yasnaya Polyana. We had our lunch at the roadside and tarried so long that the house itself was closed by the time we arrived. The grounds, however, were open. We admired the huge tree under which was the seat to which Tolstoy came each morning. He rang the bell (which was still hanging from a branch) as a signal for the villagers to come to him if they were in need of advice.

Among Luria's considerable photographic equipment he had a polaroid camera, which was then a novelty in the U.S.S.R. Some evenings he suggested we should go out and amuse ourselves with this camera. We passed through the Kremlin gates into an open space where people strolled leisurely. Luria would approach a stranger, photograph him, and then present him with a print. This caused immense excitement, and soon we were surrounded by an eager crowd asking to be photographed. Luria thoroughly enjoyed himself until his film was exhausted. Then he would say: "Let us go".

As well as his lecture-tours in Great Britain and the U.S.A., Luria enjoyed travel throughout Eastern Europe and Asia. As a keen photographer, he was able to perpetuate his experiences. He had recently trodden "the golden road" to Samarkand and Trebizond, and he did his best to persuade me to do the same. But I preferred to stay in Moscow and work. A recent holiday had taken him through Finland and the North-West Territories of the U.S.S.R. The following year he went to Siberia. I could see from the photographs he showed me the considerable beauty of those regions.

Another visit of his had been to China, and he returned with much chinoiserie, some of which he generously gave to me. Amongst those gifts was a long scroll on which was written a poem in Chinese characters. Much later I used the scroll as one of my tests of visual perception and imagery, powers of retention, speed of performance, feature-analysis, and the direction of the ocular movements of search. Luria would have chuckled to know how I was utilising his present to me.

Unfortunately it was not possible, because of my other commitments, to stay for more than a month. My return journey was remarkable in that the passenger in front of me, a Russian travelling to Canada, dropped dead. I tried without success to resuscitate him, so the plane was diverted to Copenhagen and the dead passenger taken off, complete with death certificate from me.

Like F.M.R. Walshe, Luria was constantly engaged in writing; almost compulsively so. Many of his major works were translated into English, though often after a gap of some years.

There are also two smaller works which are minor classics. Luria was reviving the traditions of romantic science when he wrote *The Mind of a Mnemonist* (1968) and *The Man With a Shattered World* (1972). He had discussed with me the subject matter of the latter book when I was with him in Moscow. In due course, he sent me a copy with this dedication: "For my dear, dear friend, Dr. Macdonald Critchley, who invented the title of this book, with affection and esteem".

Luria and I continued to correspond, and my next visit to Moscow gave me an opportunity to meet him again. The occasion was in October 1965, when the Medical Pilgrims went to Leningrad and Moscow. I lunched with Professor Luria, in the company of Professor Sarkisov and Professor Anoukhin. The following day the Medical Pilgrims dined at the British Embassy. After dinner, I took Dr. Oliver, the Embassy doctor, to visit Luria, before catching the midnight sleeper to Leningrad.

When a large Congress of Soviet neurologists and psychiatrists met in Moscow in 1969, I attended as President of the

World Federation of Neurology. Luria and his wife met me at the airport, and they invited me to dine in their apartment that evening. He had remembered that I like fish, for the delicious *ling* was served. It was a cosy family party with his wife, daughter and son-in-law present. On this occasion he showed me the magnificent insignia of the Order of Lenin, with which he had been invested. I was to be in Moscow for less than a week and had a busy schedule, but Luria graciously put at my disposal his car and his driver, so that I was able to do some sight-seeing outside the city. Another memorable evening was spent watching the Bolshoi Ballet give a marvellous performance of "Don Quixote".

I last saw Luria in London during one of his lecture-tours, when, unfortunately, he was taken ill and he became a patient of mine. I continued to prescribe medication for him which was not then available in the U.S.S.R., but did not see him again. On publication, he sent me copies of his books, and we wrote regularly to each other. He died on 14th August 1977.

Many obituaries appeared, for Luria's influence on psychological thinking had been profound and far-reaching. The tributes were laudatory, but scarcely one of them gave much idea of the man himself. The same can be said about his unconventional autobiography which was published posthumously in 1979 under the title *The Making of Mind. A Personal Account of Soviet Psychology*. The book essentially deals with Luria's career, and there is little that is self-revelatory. He was a modest and very private individual.

One obituarist wrote that Luria "... was not a happy man. He had the perfectly developed social automatisms of an easy-going man, but there was much bitterness". That is not the Luria I knew. I never saw a hint of bitterness, and I never heard him speak in derogatory terms of anyone or anything, whatever the setbacks or interruptions that may have occurred in his career.

I have made no attempt to catalogue Luria's abundant contributions to the literature. Nor have I sought to identify his great impact on neuropsychology throughout the world. Oliver Zangwill did this admirably (*Trends in Neuroscience*, 1981, vol. 4).

Luria was a most stimulating colleague, whose ideas and methods of examination were refreshingly original and exciting. His enthusiasm was contagious, and no one who worked with him could be impervious to his dynamism. "No pyramids set off his memories but the eternal substance of his greatness".

1884–1966
Georg H. Monrad-Krohn

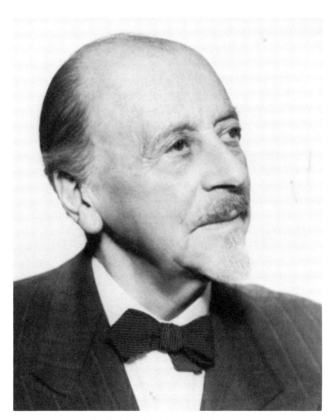

GEORG H. MONRAD-KROHN

Courtesy of the Royal College of Physicians, London.

Twenty-five years ago one commonly witnessed something of a ritual at the conclusion of every neurological meeting in Europe. Even before the applause had died down and the Chairman had time to intervene, Professor Henner of Prague would leap to his feet like a jack-in-the-box. Standing as immobile as a ramrod, he would bark out a staccato formal vote of thanks. With equal abruptness, he would resume his seat.

Later in the day, perhaps towards the end of the official dinner, Monrad-Krohn would, with exquisite grace, stand and, to the delight of everyone present, beam benignly at the company. Pink-cheeked, flaxen-haired and smiling, he would adjust his monocle, finger his bow-tie, and proceed to his congratulatory address. He did not stare fixedly ahead like an automaton, nor did he direct his remarks to the ceiling. He seemed to be addressing everyone individually. His words came out with fluency and grace, whether in French, German or English. Indeed, his command of the last-named was, if anything, too good. None could fault his pronunciation. Those severe custodians of the Queen's English, the five vowels, had been mastered. The other tricky phonemes, the terminal plural sibilant; the ensnaring "l" and "r"; the difficult fricative "th"; and the gutturally modified bilabial voiced spirant "w"; Monrad-Krohn had conquered all these linguistic traps for foreigners. Just why his English was "too good" will be told later.

He was at his best when proposing the health of the ladies present at the banquet. There was a runner-up in this *genre,* however, namely Schaltenbrand of Würzburg. Whereas Schaltenbrand was serious, even a little ponderous, Monrad-Krohn was light-hearted and *pétillant*. Undoubtedly he was a ladies' man, a *coqueluche des femmes*.

Monrad-Krohn was Norwegian, and surely the most elegant, dandified Viking there ever was; the most urbane of Norsemen. Kim Borg said that Scandinavians have a strange feeling of being at once outside of Europe and part of it. Monrad-Krohn was undoubtedly a European.

Born in 1884 in the attractive Hanseatic port of Bergen, he attended its University and qualified in medicine, being the fourth in direct line of apothecaries and doctors. As a student, he won a gold medal for an essay on the conduction of nerve-impulses in the heart. His next step was to visit London and secure the necessary diploma in order to practice medicine in England. He remained in London for five years, from 1913 to 1917.

Armed with this British qualification, he applied successfully for the post of Resident Medical Officer to the Hospital for Epilepsy and Paralysis, Maida Vale. He also regularly visited the clinics at the National Hospital, Queen Square. Thus he learned his neurology. That was not all. He sat the formidable examination which entitled him to Membership of the Royal College of Physicians. He was also awarded the Gaskell silver medal for 1917 for work in psychiatry.

Before returning to Norway, he visited Paris and attended both the Salpêtrière and the Bicêtre, thus becoming the pupil of Pierre Marie and of Babinski.

Monrad-Krohn and I met frequently. He often visited England, and he never failed to call in at the National Hospital. No doubt he met his publishers regularly, for he was one of their best-sellers. Like every British neurologist of my generation, I had studied with approval his *Blue Book of Neurology*, as Norwegian students called it (*Clinical Examination of the Nervous System*). It had originally appeared, in English, in 1921, and it ran to 12 editions and many re-writings, and had been translated into several languages.

In my visits to Europe, I seemed constantly to bump into

Monrad-Krohn. He probably said the same about me. When I became Dean of the Institute of Neurology, I arranged for him to give guest lectures at the National Hospital in 1947, and again in 1952.

He published a large number of articles, contributing to the neurological journals of many countries. Though his literary output was considerable, he betrayed a certain repetitiousness. He had two or three abiding interests in neurology which he discussed again and again. Like his pioneer fellow-townsman, Dr. G.H.A. Hansen, he had considerable experience of leprosy, and wrote much on the neurological complications of that disease. For this work he was made a Chevalier of the Légion d'Honneur. His interest in the various reflex phenomena was profound, though the Bechterew school of reflexology did not attract him.

Monrad-Krohn was particularly interested in the vagaries of the abdominal responses in neurological disorders. The differing degrees of difficulty in their elicitation; their "inversion"; the relationship between the abdominal and the cremasteric reflexes—such were some of the questions which he pursued with all the acumen of a dedicated clinician. He emphasized the distinction between the superficial reflex elicited by stroking with a pin, and a pericostal-abdominal contraction evoked by tapping the costal margin. The phenomena of exhaustion and of facilitation of the abdominal responses were carefully described.

In a paper published in 1919, he reported the results of a field study carried out in a strenuous 50 kilometre ski-race lasting $4\frac{3}{4}$ hours. There were 49 contestants, and he noted the state of their knee-jerks before and immediately after this exercise. In all but two cases, the knee-jerks became markedly diminished.

Facial palsy was another interest. He realised that Gowers had observed a dissociation between voluntary and emotional facial movements following central lesions; and that this phenomenon had been overlooked by almost everyone else. At times, he noticed, the paralysed side of the patient's face might display exaggerated movements under the influence of emotion.

Two other neurological interests were shared by us, namely speech-disorders and blindness.

Visitors to Scandinavia notice that people there speak with a conspicuous lilt, and the melody of their speech differs somewhat according to whether they are Danes, Swedes, or Norwegians. Monrad-Krohn spoke of this tonal quality as "prosody", and he labelled it "the third element" in speech. He had noticed that this speech-melody might alter or even disappear altogether, after a stroke involving the dominant hemisphere. A dysprosody was most likely to follow a mild or resolving aphasia. The first patient to arouse his attention to this phenomenon was a Norwegian lady, who found during her convalescence after a transient cerebrovascular accident that she was cold-shouldered by shopkeepers and by strangers to whom she had spoken. It was at the time of the German occupation of Norway, and she eventually realised that she was being mistaken for a foreigner. Monrad-Krohn wrote many articles on this subject.

In his later papers dealing with "the third element of speech" he also drew attention to the occurrence of "prosodic grunts", which, though inarticulate, were nonetheless meaningful. He might well have said with Thomas Shadwell: "Words may be false and full of art, while grunts are the natural language of the heart".

Monrad-Krohn has been described as a somewhat old-fashioned neurologist. I believe that this is unfair. Certainly he was not a neuroscientist but essentially a clinician, which perhaps entails qualities that are more elusive, more difficult to acquire, and more directly in line with the making of a good doctor.

His interest in the blind was more limited. He addressed medical societies in both Trondheim and in Bergen in 1959 on the question whether sightless people possess a sixth sense which assists them in avoiding obstacles. His paper appeared in the *Nord. Med.*, 1962:67, but was never published in English.

Earlier I stated that Monrad-Krohn's command of English was, if anything "too good". The fact is that he spoke with great fluency the English of an earlier generation. His ready use of colloquial or slang expressions was out of date. The adjectives "ripping" and "topping" came readily to his tongue, in the same way as the interjection "By Jove". As Hazlitt said, "Words, like clothes, get old-fashioned . . . when they have been for some time laid aside".

Monrad-Krohn must have spoken English well before he left Bergen, one of his first tasks in London being to sit the M.R.C.S. and L.R.C.P. diplomas in 1913.

On his many subsequent visits to London he stayed at the Royal Automobile Club in Pall Mall. There was an occasion when I arranged to meet him there just after lunch. I put myself and my car at his disposal, telling him that I had arranged for us to dine that evening at The Mitre, Hampton Court. In the meantime, I told him, I would drive him wherever he liked in London or in the country. He thought for a while and then asked diffidently whether I would take him to Bexley in Kent. I assured him that that was simple, and that we could go there via Greenwich and Blackheath and return by a leisurely roundabout route to Hampton Court for dinner. He was delighted, and he explained that during his five-year sojourn in London he had taken a locum job at Bexley Mental Hospital. It was obvious that his visit there that day had evoked old memories of a romantic nature.

In 1953 he told me he had received financial support from the Norwegian Guild of Shipowners, and asked me to make a two-week lecture tour in Bergen and Oslo. September in Norway is delightful, and I discovered the paintings of Edvard Munch. Being interested in self-portraiture, I found Munch's work especially significant. There were portraits of himself at various ages, in sickness as well as in health. To anyone studying disorders of the body-image, Munch's paintings are particularly valuable.

In Oslo, where Monrad-Krohn occupied the Chair of Neurology, I met the charming but strict ritual of the dinner-table, and warm hospitality on all sides. I was honoured by being elected to the Norwegian Academy of Science and Arts. I went back to Bergen, where Professor Refsum then occupied the Chair of Neurology, in order to return to England by sea.

The neurological pioneers of the 19th century, on the whole, lived in circumstances of serenity and calm. Not so their sons and grandsons. Most of these endured one world war, others two. Some had to survive harsh political regimes. Many somehow managed to carry on teaching, to do research, and to practice under the hostile scrutiny of an alien occupying force. I have known many of them; usually they remained silent on the subject. Monrad-Krohn was different.

In July 1946, just over a year after the surrender of his country's invaders, he visited Newcastle upon Tyne and lectured to the medical school of the University of Durham about the life of Norwegians during the occupation. He said that during the months immediately following the German invasion, the Norwegian Army, ill-armed and unprepared, put up a brave but hopeless resistance. There was a shortage of insulin and also of anaesthetic drugs. Medical students made secret forays across the Swedish border and returned with the necessary supplies.

From the Ruhr came Terboven, reputed to have been a fraudulent bank-clerk. He was installed as *Reichskommissar*. He had a pathological hatred of intellectuals and academics; the University of Oslo came under his power. Even more hostile was a Norwegian-born academic, "X". He proposed that prominent German professors should be invited to give lectures in Oslo, but Monrad-Krohn would not agree. Under the German Minister of Health was a former assistant of Monrad-Krohn's ... "a good enough neurologist but hardly qualified for his job". He once denounced his former chief to one of the leaders of the N.S. (*National Sammling*), a minority group of Fascist-minded young Norwegians established by Quisling before the war.

On 1st January 1941 the Dean of the Faculty of Medicine retired, and Monrad-Krohn was appointed to succeed him. The Germans then dismissed the Rector and replaced him by "X". Oslo was by now under martial law. The former Dean and a number of distinguished professors were held as hostages and two were shot as non-collaborators.

Within the medical faculty there was a particularly dangerous traitor, Professor "Y". He found he could not cope with the many problems that beset the University and so a Pro-Rector, a former polar explorer was appointed. Although he was nominally a member of the N.S. party, on the whole, according to Monrad-Krohn, he was a decent man in his dealings with the University.

In the autumn of 1942, "X" demanded that 16 N.S. members should be admitted as medical students. The Dean and his committee refused to do so, and Monrad-Krohn was summoned to appear before Quisling. The meeting was a stormy one, but, after threats that "heads would roll", Quisling suddenly changed his mind. None of the N.S. students was admitted.

Eventually the authorities closed the University and hundreds of the students were arrested. Many were sent to Germany. Fearing that the medical faculty might re-open under German and N.S. domination, Monrad-Krohn converted the lecture theatres in the hospitals into wards for patients.

Their troubles ended on 7th May 1945, when General Böhme, Commander-in-Chief of the enemy forces, broadcast the surrender. Norwegian troops took over strategic points throughout the country; collaborators were arrested and Quisling, among others, was executed.

This account of academic life in Norway during the German occupation is based entirely upon Monrad-Krohn's lecture. The topic was never referred to in conversation either with Monrad-Krohn himself or with any of his colleagues whom I met from time to time.

My last meeting with Monrad-Krohn was in 1961, on the occasion of the International Congress of Neurology in Rome.

As far as I can remember, I do not think he attended the next Congress in Vienna in 1965.

Monrad-Krohn died in 1966. His last photographs show that he had grown a beard of formal cut, not the untidy, straggling beard of the slovenly aged, but a neatly trimmed, dandified growth. He must have retained intact his *image de soi* well into his 80s.

Thus passed a personality from the world's neurological scene, one who is remembered with great affection and who is much missed by those who were fortunate enough to have known him and to have been taught by him.

1889–1947
George Riddoch

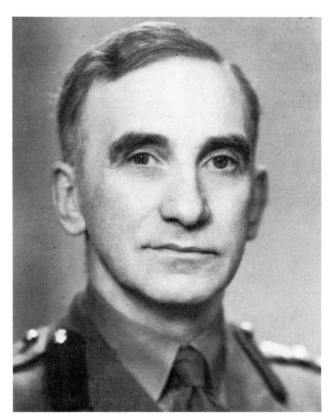

GEORGE RIDDOCH

Courtesy of the Institute of Neurology, London.

How many neurologists today are familiar with the name and work of George Riddoch? Yet in his day he had the largest neurological practice in London and medical students at the London Hospital revered him for his teaching skill, his friendliness and his outrageous sense of fun. Throughout his comparatively short life he was driven by a vaulting ambition to succeed, but the expected accolades and official recognition eluded him.

He was born in Keith, a small town in Banffshire, in the north of Scotland. After his schooldays at Robert Gordon's College, Aberdeen, he received his medical training in the ancient university in that city. His career was a brilliant one. He qualified in 1913 with first-class honours, and four years later he obtained his M.D. degree with the highest distinction.

Riddoch attracted the notice of Dr. Ashley Mackintosh, a wise physician with an interest in nervous disorders. Like so many northerners, Riddoch knew that the principal prizes were to be found in the metropolis. Just before the first World War, he was appointed a house physician to the West End Hospital for Nervous Disorders (or the Nervous Hospital for West End Disorders, as it has been dubbed). There he much impressed Sir James Purves Stewart, that lone but successful figure on the fringe of the neurological clique.

Riddoch's first great opportunity came when, as a Captain in the Royal Army Medical Corps, he was posted to the Empire Hospital for Officers in Vincent's Square, London. In charge was the eminent Henry Head, who took an immediate liking to his keen junior officer. A fruitful collaboration followed in research into the effects of spinal cord injuries. The various reflex phenomena were described and interpreted along physiological lines as promulgated by Sherrington. Dysfunction of the bladder and bowel was closely studied, and several papers were published in *Brain*, including one in which they described the so-called "mass-reflex". Riddoch later wrote a valuable article dealing with visuoperceptual disorders resulting from war wounds of the occipital lobe. His paper on visual disorientation in homonymous half-fields (*Brain*, 1935) was an important one. Unfortunately he did not continue this work with any other researches into disorders of vision.

In 1916 he married Margaret Ledingham, a charming and sympathetic lady who was also from Aberdeen. There were three children.

Some time during his career, Riddoch visited Paris; he became a life-long friend of Professor Jean Lhermitte. Details of this period are obscure, but it is certain that, after 1923, Riddoch scarcely ever left London; he seemed to concentrate upon building up a medical practice.

No doubt because of his wartime association with Henry Head, who had been Physician to the London Hospital, Riddoch gained entry to the staff. Shortly after the war, a "medical unit" was set up at that hospital and Riddoch was elected as an assistant to that unit. In 1924 he became a supernumerary assistant physician to the London Hospital, there being no vacancy at the time.

Meanwhile, in 1919 he had become a Physician to the Hospital for Epilepsy and Paralysis, Maida Vale. Here he impressed Campbell Thompson, the senior physician, with his abilities. Riddoch resigned this appointment in 1924 on being elected to the staff of the National Hospital, Queen Square, though not without some opposition. The translation from Maida Vale to Queen Square was the first of several migrations of the staff, ceasing only when the two hospitals became officially amalgamated.

George Riddoch was striking in appearance though short in stature. Unlike so many Scots from the northeast area which is rich in Scandinavian stock, he was a Celt, raven-haired, dark-eyed, and an aquiline nose. Shortly before I first met him, I had seen Galsworthy's play *Loyalties* in the West End. I was immediately reminded of the character Ferdinand de Levis, as played by Ernest Milton.

Riddoch's speech was pure Doric, attractively laced with such Scottishisms as "wee" and "bawbies". The diminutive suffix "ie" abounded in his talk, and was an important constituent of his charm.

As a practising neurologist, Riddoch showed two principal facets. In the first place, he amassed a considerable clientèle for patients found him optimistic and comforting. Referring doctors were impressed by the firmness of his opinions as to diagnosis and treatment. Towards his patients he exuded attentiveness, reassurance and compassion. He emanated confidence and understanding. When Riddoch died, his junior colleague, Russell Brain, repeatedly referred in his tribute to his humanity.

Riddoch's other interest lay in teaching, particularly undergraduates, with whom he was vastly popular. He was unhesitatingly didactic. In his diagnoses there was no question of "might be" or "possibly"; the patient before him was always "a clear case" of this or that disorder. But his dogmatism was often more convincing than the facts would warrant. His students relished his positive assertions, which made neurology less of a mystery than it was reputed to be. He was a constant source of friendly mimicry, with his pronounced accent and his many mannerisms. Chief among the latter was his habit of wiping his nose with the back of his hand from right to left, like a schoolboy who had lost his handkerchief. This action commonly heralded something particularly important that he was about to say.

Compared with most other neurologists, Riddoch did not write a great deal. He was, however, deeply interested in the phenomena associated with phantom limbs, and his probing interrogations brought to light many points of great interest about which some patients were too embarrassed to speak.

He was also concerned in the problem of central pain. In 1938 he and I together wrote a paper on this topic which was to be read in Paris at the June meeting of the Société de Neurologie. Much of the writing was done in my dining room. While I sat scribbling, he paced up and down the floor, now and again being inspired to utter a sentence—not a technique to be recommended. In time the paper was finished, and it was sent to the Berlitz School for translation into the French of Flaubert and Maupassant.

In Paris the question arose as to which of us should read the text. We tossed a coin. Riddoch was to read the paper and I was to answer any questions that arose during the discussion. Mine was the more hazardous job, so I carefully seated myself next to a French friend who spoke fluent English.

Riddoch was masterly, the accent of Aberdeen blending with his French in an attractive harmony. When the applause ended, someone in the audience asked a question. The reply was simple, a straightforward negative. For me to leap to my feet with a firm "non" struck me as risky, so I asked my bilingual neighbour to answer for me. He agreed, but it took twelve minutes of rapid verbiage to do so.

That evening there was to be a banquet at Maxim's Restaurant. Neurologists from all over Europe would be there. We suspected that one of us might be called upon to say a few words. Riddoch and I adjourned to the lobby, and on hotel writing paper we concocted a speech in sixth-form schoolboy French. Each of us pocketed a copy. Thus prepared, we sat down to our feast at a table glistening with crystal and silver and a small posy before each guest. At the end, coffee was served. Riddoch and I exchanged interrogatory glances, but before either of us could get up, Purves Stewart, who had been out of our sight, rose to his feet and delivered a characteristically unctuous speech on behalf of British neurology. So Riddoch and I were spared.

The high-spot of the evening came when Professor Ley of Brussels arose. "Before me", he proclaimed, "I see a beautiful rose." With deliberation he raised the flower to his nostrils and solemnly sniffed it. He went on. "I regard this little blossom as a symbol. A symbol", and here his voice rose, "*de l'amitié Franco-Belge!*" The applause was tremendous, and the evening ended upon that satisfactory note.

One of Georgie Riddoch's most endearing roles was that of a raconteur of Rabelaisian tales. In this way he would buttonhole a colleague and proceed upon what was obviously going to be a "chestnut", familiar since boyhood. But he could not be halted, and, as he proceeded, he began to laugh and his articulation faltered; tears ran down his cheeks, but, mopping his eyes with his handkerchief, he struggled on. The performance never lost its appeal.

In the late 1930s, Riddoch bought a country property at Bourne End, beside the River Thames. He rested here at weekends if he was not too busy. I can recall Georgie at the end of the garden, fishing rod in hand, practising the art of casting a line. Only too often, however, his peace was disturbed by urgent calls to see a patient.

Riddoch was tireless in the care of his old chief Henry Head, who, since retirement, had developed Parkinson's disease. Head refused all medical treatment, fearing that the drugs then available might blunt the sharp edge of his intellect. Riddoch arranged for a team to give his patient intensive physiotherapy throughout the whole day. Henry Head also found temporary benefit from the vibration resulting from car rides over rough country.

With the declaration of the Second World War in September 1939, Riddoch became a consultant in neurology to the Emergency Medical Service. He continued to live at his house in Devonshire Place, while visiting hospitals anywhere in England. His duties did not preclude his continuing private practice, but the burden was great and obviously fatiguing. Later in the war he was also made a consultant to the Army at home, with the rank of Brigadier. Despite these extra duties, he still lived at home. The work-load was heavy, for his duties also included much travel and attendance at many inter-service committees.

Riddoch's health began to suffer. Migrainous headaches occurred only too often, and, later, symptoms of a peptic ulcer developed. He was seen to resort to analgesics for his head pain, and these aggravated his dyspepsia, necessitating another type of pill. This alternation of pill-taking went on throughout every day. When particularly tired he would listen to music in his drawing room, a measure which brought him relaxation even though temporarily so. He was especially refreshed by listening to Delius, that curt and crippled artist who, I believe, had once been his patient.

As consulting neurologist to the Army, it was one of his duties to interview Rudolf Hess, whose behaviour in custody was causing concern. Was he psychotic? hysterical? a malingerer? The problem increased when Hess tried to commit suicide by throwing himself into the well of a lofty stairway. The result was a fractured femur. Later still, Hess was transferred to Europe, and, before the Nuremberg trials began, a high-level medical examination was required. Riddoch flew to Germany in the company of the consultant in psychiatry to the Army and also the President of the Royal College of Physicians, each of whom disliked the other two.

Towards the end of the war I saw a good deal of Riddoch, and we often dined together at the Athenaeum. Over and above his gastric symptoms, he showed striking mood-swings; sometimes he was excited and hyperactive. There was talk of an impending National Health Service, in which Riddoch became deeply interested. Often he would join me at the Club carrying a bundle of documents, and throughout the meal he would read this or that paper. Then, looking round the dining room he would espy at another table a Ministry official or a senior Civil Servant. Riddoch would interrupt his dinner and accost that person to discuss some point of concern to him. These interruptions might occur three or four times, but he would nevertheless contrive to finish eating before I did, because he was a very rapid eater.

Matters came to a dramatic head one morning at the War Office while he was examining a patient. He was seized with an intense pain in his upper abdomen. Helped into a taxi, he was driven to the London Hospital where a bed was found for him, I believe in the Nurses' Home. En route, so he told me, he debated whether he had sustained a coronary infarction or a perforated peptic ulcer. He decided, correctly, in favour of the latter.

He was operated on without delay, and two or three days later I went to visit him at the hospital. I asked the Hall Porter in which ward I would find Brigadier Riddoch. I was told he was at a committee meeting. "But", I expostulated, "it isn't long since he was operated on". "Can't help that" was the reply. "That's where he is. I'll tell him you're here. Please wait in the consultants' sitting room". Five minutes later the door opened and Riddoch, fully dressed, came to greet me at a run. In so doing he stumbled over a waste-paper basket, spilling its contents on to the floor. Riddoch dropped on to his hands and knees to retrieve each piece of rubbish, until I almost forcibly restrained him.

The manic phase was followed by a deep depression. When we met again about 10 days later, he told me that a second and more serious operation was necessary. He was dreading it, and feared returning to hospital. My suggestion was that he should at once take a holiday in Aberdeen and, if he experienced any abdominal symptoms, he should consult his life-long friend, the able surgeon Willy Anderson. Riddoch's face lit up and he eagerly agreed to the idea. But it was not to be.

The next and last time I saw George Riddoch was at the doorway of the National Hospital. "I have got to go into the London tomorrow", he said. "I didn't go to Aberdeen". Two highly skilled surgeons operated, and the surgery proceeded without a hitch. There were no post-operative complications. All had apparently gone well, but Riddoch simply did not rally.

As the saying is, "He turned his face to the wall" and died 4 days later on 24th October 1947.

Riddoch's story was, in some ways, a sad one. He should have borne in mind the warning given by William Osler to the students of Yale . . . "One of the saddest of life's tragedies is the wreckage of the career of the young collegian by hurry, bustle, bustle and tension—the human machine driven day and night, as no sensible fellow would use his motor". Georgie had come to London as a *Wunderkind* from the Highlands, full of drive and enthusiasm. He was, however, like a juggler with too many balls in the air. So many aspects of his neurological career appealed to him, that he did not know where to concentrate his abilities. Investigative neurology attracted him. As a great teacher he might have written the standard manual of neurology, for such textbooks were lacking in the 1920s. Committee work, too, he enjoyed, and he could have become a wise medical administrator like his junior colleague, Russell Brain. But most seductive of all and immediate in its financial returns, was the lure of private practice. Although Georgie would have liked to fill all these roles, it was not possible.

Did he make the right choice? Who can say. Those doctors who have concentrated most of their working lives on seeing patients, do not leave tangible evidence of their work and are soon forgotten. But multitudes of sick patients were the beneficiaries, as were generations of students.

1903–1975
E. Graeme Robertson

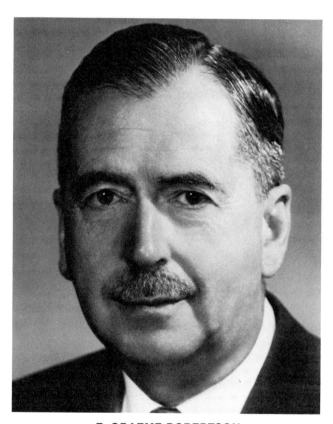

E. GRAEME ROBERTSON

In the first third of this present century, it was the rule that there should be three resident medical officers at the National Hospital, Queen Square. The last to be appointed was the junior, and he moved up the scale as vacancies arose. The most senior bore the title of Resident Medical Officer. The term of office was three years. Accommodation was good, for each resident had his own sitting room in addition to his bedroom. It is understandable that such an opportunity was a highly prized one and rarely, if ever, was there an application from one who was not making neurology his career.

The manner in which the House Physicians were allocated to the Chiefs, that is, the Honorary Physicians, was unusual. The most senior House Physician (the Resident Medical Officer) had the privilege of choosing which of the eleven members of the staff he would serve. The next senior House Physician had the second choice, and the junior House Physician was assigned to whomever was left.

The House Physicians took it in turns to act as House Surgeon.

The rules of chance ordained that at times there would be in residence three would-be neurologists of exceptional ability, whose subsequent careers were outstanding.

Such was the case in the period 1928–1931, when such eminent figures as Ritchie Russell, Denny-Brown, Denis Brinton, S.P. Meadows, Douglas Buchanan, J.St.C. Elkington and Graeme Robertson were in residence.

Graeme Robertson came to Queen Square from Melbourne. He was quite unlike the average Englishman's conception of an Australian. He was not tall and muscular; he was no athlete; his voice was quiet, and his accent impeccable—well, almost.

Everyone liked this quiet Australian. He and Denny-Brown collaborated in research projects, but perhaps his closest friend was Brinton—future neurologist to the National Hospital and to St. Mary's Hospital, where for many years he served as Dean.

In those early days I did not see a great deal of Graeme; he was never my House Physician. His great guru was Gordon Holmes, whom he understandably held in the highest esteem and affection. When Holmes retired and went to live in Farnham, Graeme Robertson never failed to call on him on his numerous visits to England.

I saw much more of Graeme Robertson after he left England to take up an appointment as Assistant Physician to the Royal Melbourne Hospital in 1934. Ten years later, a special department of neurology was created with Graeme in charge.

His outlook on neurology was international, and he kept in close personal touch with his teachers in London; he regularly attended neurological congresses in North America and in Europe.

Thus it came about that I saw a great deal of Graeme; my contacts were reestablished by my two-weeks visits to Melbourne in 1953 and in 1967. On the latter occasion, Graeme Robertson was President of the Second Asian-Australasian Congress of Neurology. He organised this polyglot symposium with considerable but inconspicuous efficiency and tact, an achievement which many of us confidently expected would be officially recognised; in that we were disappointed. As Edmund Burke grimly remarked, "A king may make a nobleman, but not a gentleman". Graeme had done that for himself.

Graeme Robertson was an excellent all-round neurologist with a busy practice in Collings Street. As his colleague, R.S. Cooper, asserted, Graeme was fortunate in living at the right time, what he called "The Golden Age of Neurology". His quiet understanding of the difficulties of his patients, his essential integrity, were qualities soon recognised and widely appreciated. As a neurologist he mastered one difficult technique with such care and skill that he became surely the world authority upon pneumoencephalography.

It may seem odd that this intrusive and unpleasant procedure, part surgical, part radiological, should have attracted his attention. Perhaps he had seen this test performed so badly that he felt called upon to perfect the technique while rendering it as little distressing as possible. He wrote at least two monographs upon this subject, in 1941 and 1957. The latter is a classic and a second edition appeared in 1967. His contribution entitled "Investigations of Intracranial Tumours by Pneumoencephalography" appeared in Volume 16 of *The Handbook of Clinical Neurology* (Vinken & Bruyn), and extended over 80 pages with 125 illustrations.

Perhaps there was in pneumoencephalography a challenge that called on all his perfectionist ideals, as well as photographic skills.

In 1950, along with seven others including, inter alia, Leonard Cox, Kenneth Noad and Eric Susman, he founded the Australian Association of Neurologists. In 1963 the Association issued its attractive annual *Clinical and Experimental Neurology*. It is difficult to avoid the belief that Graeme was the instigator of this Society. He was the second elected President of the Royal Australasian College of Physicians as well as a Vice-President of the World Federation of Neurology.

The Association of Australian Neurologists has grown *pari passu* with the great prestige of the discipline as obtains today in Australia. *Si monumentum requiris circumspice.* There is now an annual Graeme Robertson lectureship.

Graeme's principal hobby was photography, not of persons or places but almost exclusively of cast-iron gateways, railings, verandas and the like. His skill was considerable, and he became an international expert. In connection with his hobby of architectural photography, he published large tomes dealing with the verandas of Melbourne, Sydney, Tasmania, New Orleans and New York—11 volumes in all, each one a masterpiece and definitive in scope. What an achievement!

But Graeme was more than an illustrator of 19th century ironwork. He researched the subject thoroughly, and in time became the world's authority. He was made an honorary member of the Friends of Cast-Iron Architecture in the United States. He was also the President of the National Gallery of Victoria Society; and a member of the National Trust of Australia (Victoria). Graeme and his daughter, Joan, collaborated in the preparation of the 11th volume, and in the introduction wrote how an interest in cast-iron enlivens a walk in many cities, tempting one to explore areas which might otherwise have been overlooked. How many can boast of having written the definitive monograph in their own field as well as producing the supreme book on their hobby?

Like so many other neurologists, Graeme was an eccentric, but an engaging, amiable one, the acme of worldly innocence. He travelled extensively, but always seemed to be a little lost, hazy about the date—though not disorientated in time to the extent that Geoffrey Jefferson was. Graeme seemed at times to be dubious as to the place in which he currently found himself. His luggage would go astray; he would lose things; his hotel arrangements were muddled. But wherever he appeared there were always friends who came to his rescue, providing him with counsel, sustenance and accommodation—even the key of the door, so that he could come and go as his whim ordained. He seemed so helpless and yet so calm that his friends became Samaritans. His colleagues' wives were particularly touched, their motherly instincts invariably being aroused.

Once I ran into him in New Orleans, where he was busy photographing the cast-iron work so characteristic of the French Quarter. He had set up his camera with great deliberation in the rue Royale, taken photometric readings, put his light-meter down beside him on the curb and buried his head beneath the cloth. When he emerged, the picture taken, the apparatus had disappeared. At great expense he bought a replacement in Chicago. A few days later we were both in Greenwich Village— I in search of antiquarian bookshops, he looking for cast-iron verandas. The scenario repeated itself. The camera on its stand, the light-meter on the pavement, his eyes busy focusing. A successful photograph was taken, and so was his light-meter.

In Tasmania on one occasion, we found ourselves late at night locked out of the Hobart Club. There was no night-porter and Graeme had forgotten to take the key. We achieved entry by forcing open a window.

Behind his mask of unworldliness, Graeme was a shrewd and scholarly person. As H.V. Pritchett wrote, "People are always larger than they appear to be. There's more to be said about them than one thinks. You have to find out what this is . . .".

Graeme Robertson was a great collector of early Australiana, and his study was filled with ancient maps, manuscripts, pictures, old books and artefacts. His colleagues still talk about a historical lecture he delivered dealing with Melbourne in 1855, entitled "Carriages at Eleven; or a buggy-ride into the past".

He also had considerable taste in antique furniture. When I was in Melbourne, Graeme once took me to a house belonging to Keith Murdoch. The contents were to be auctioned the following day. One of the most conspicuous items was a huge kidney-shaped desk, a most unusual and handsome piece of furniture. I asked Graeme if he was interested, but he made no reply. Two days later I read in the local newspaper details of the sale. I saw that the desk had been sold for a large sum to a Collings Street physician. I showed this to Graeme, who looked slightly ill at ease but who then invited me to his consulting room. There, occupying about four-fifths of the available space, leaving just enough room for two chairs, stood the Murdoch desk. Before I had time to offer my congratulations, with some emotion Graeme told me that the first patient he had seen after the desk had arrived was a man with G.P.I. He came in with his hat on, smoking a cigar. When Graeme discreetly protested, the patient stubbed out the lighted cigar on the surface of the famous desk.

Modesty tempered the satisfaction Graeme must have felt towards the end of his career. However, we remember him for not only putting neurology on the map in Australia, but for his unique artistic achievements.

His terminal illness slowly but inexorably gained ground, and, to his great disappointment, prevented him in March 1975 from attending the celebrations at the Charing Cross Hospital which marked the 100th anniversary of the birth of his mentor, Gordon Holmes. Graeme died on Christmas Day, 1975.

1864–1939
James S. Risien Russell

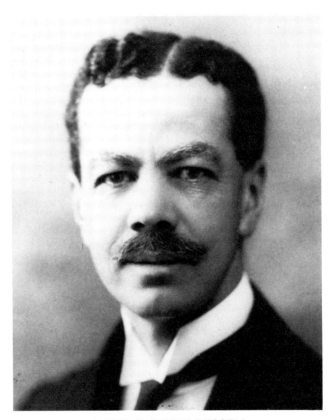

JAMES S. RISIEN RUSSELL

Courtesy of the Institute of Neurology, London.

In those distant student days, I knew but little of the *dramatis personae* of neurology. Friedreich I knew about because of his ataxia. Brown-Séquard, too, was vaguely familiar. Perhaps the best-known was Erb, largely because my teacher took pains to pronounce the name in correct German and not Bristol-fashion, as we students were apt to do. There was, however, one British neurologist I had heard of, a contemporary figure who was a spectacular teacher and who had an enormous practice. This was J.S. Risien Russell.

I first met him when I was an applicant for the post of house physician, calling upon him at his immense corner house in Wimpole Street. The furniture was in excellent taste, elegant and, no doubt, costly. His appearance, however, was somewhat of a surprise. He was a small, dapper, youthful-looking man, though he must have been almost 60 years of age. He had close-cropped, curly, jet-black hair, a small greyish moustache, and a dark skin. He was impeccably dressed in a brown suit, and his small feet were encased in highly polished tan shoes.

The atmosphere he exuded was one of great charm and friendliness. I left the interview feeling I had discovered a warm-hearted friend, as indeed he proved to be.

Subsequently I learned that he had been born in what was then British Guiana. Apparently his father had been a man of some importance in the city of Georgetown, for a statue had been erected there in his memory.

Where Risien Russell received his schooling, I do not know. His medical education took place in Edinburgh and he qualified in 1886, later attaining his M.D. with a gold medal. Assisted by a scholarship, he carried out postgraduate studies in Paris and

Berlin. No doubt he was an eager attendant at Charcot's Tuesday demonstrations.

He became Resident Medical Officer to the National Hospital in 1888. An old, old lady once told me she had been a nurse at that hospital, and well remembered that during the Christmas Day revels a large wicker basket was dragged around the wards from which sprang Risien Russell dressed as Mephistopheles, to the delight of the patients.

During the next decade Risien Russell assisted Victor Horsley in his anatomical researches. Many were carried out in Horsley's house in Cavendish Square, the billiard room having been converted into a laboratory. They worked in collaboration upon the cerebellum and its connections, the brachial plexus, the lumbosacral plexus, and the innervation of the larynx.

He was then appointed Consulting Physician to the National Hospital, where he remained for the next 30 years. Thus, he knew intimately Hughlings Jackson, Gowers, Ferrier, Bastian and other great figures who were his colleagues. About the same time, he was elected to the consulting staff of University College Hospital, London, as Professor of Clinical Medicine and also of Forensic Medicine.

Early in the 20th century, Risien Russell wrote several important papers dealing with clinico-pathological topics. Thus, with Dr. Kingdon he gave a complete account of the nature and morbid anatomy of that entity usually referred to as Tay-Sachs disease. He wrote many chapters in Allbut and Rolleston's *System of Medicine*, using, incidentally, the unusual term "disseminate sclerosis" for what most physicians either call disseminated or else multiple sclerosis. His writings were unusually clear and polished in style.

Perhaps Risien Russell's most important contribution was the pioneer description of what British neurologists usually refer to as subacute combined degeneration of the spinal cord. This paper, which appeared in *Brain,* 1900, vol. 23, was written in association with his junior colleagues, F.E. Batten and James Collier.

Knowing something of his background, but not all, of course, I was anxious to see this great man at work. When I became a resident at Queen Square in December 1923, my opportunity came. I was warned off by the senior housemen from attending case-presentations given by members of the honorary staff, but, as a newcomer, I took a chance. Having crept into the back of the small lecture hall, I gazed in astonishment at Risien Russell demonstrating a patient with syringobulbia.

In the front row of the audience sat a huge, black doctor, who was delighted, though no doubt embarrassed, when Risien Russell directed all his remarks to him personally, continually addressing him as "my friend". To indicate that the patient's syrinx had involved the last few cranial nerves on one side, Risien addressed the black student. "When I ask this poor man to phonate", he said, turning to the patient and telling him to say 'ah', "you will observe, my friend, that the palatal elevation is oblique. And when I request him to protrude his tongue— stick out your tongue, my man—you will notice, my friend, that it deviates to one side". This was delivered in a dramatic manner, accompanied by elaborate gestures. The message was simple, but the delivery was riveting. I stifled the thought that I was in the Sunday morning market in Petticoat Lane. In fact, this was Risien Russell's last case presentation, and it was showmanship at its best. It was a most attractive, unusual performance. Never again did I see him teach students, because he did his ward-rounds without them being present.

As his House Physician, I would wait in the front hall of the hospital for his arrival. His Rolls-Royce car drove up and the chauffeur alighted to open the door for him. Risien bounded up the stairs two or three at a time, his movements being as quick as those of an athlete. As he made his way round the wards, he had a kind word of praise, or even flattery, for each patient. Each one felt buoyed up after the remarks he made smilingly, even though he never carried out a physical exami-nation. I do not usually employ the over-used word "charisma", but when applied to Risien Russell it is apt. Even a young woman with multiple sclerosis whose condition was worsening rapidly was temporarily the happier after Risien's visit. As he approached her bed, he exclaimed "My dear little lady, what a gorgeous nightdress!". His remark did more to help than all our therapeutic efforts. As is said in the Royal Navy, he could charm an anchor through a hawse-hole.

His patients were scattered throughout the hospital, and after he visited the wards other patients would say to me, "Why can't I be under the care of that nice doctor?".

Despite his failure to examine his patients, his clinical sense was spell-binding. He was the supreme exponent of instantaneous diagnosis. A story circulated that, when he was Physician-in-Charge of Outpatients, he had turned his head to glance at a newcomer being wheeled into the clinic and then said to the class, "We are now in the presence of a case of Friedreich's ataxia." No hint or intimation of the diagnosis had been given to him beforehand.

Many such split-second evaluations did I witness, and I even began to suspect that he had seen the patients before, perhaps in Wimpole Street, until an occasion when, entering John Back ward, he took one look at a patient and said, "Ah, a case of syringomyelia". "Sir", I said, "You must have seen this man before". On his denial, I asked him, "How then did you immediately know the diagnosis?". Risien smiled. "Here is a young man of 20 or 30, with wasting of his hands. The eyelid on one side is drooping, and the pupil of that eye is too small. His pain-sense must be reduced because there is a small scar of a cigarette burn between the tips of the nicotine-stained index and second fingers. What else could it be but syringo-myelia?".

This was so different from most of my chiefs, particularly Gordon Holmes who abhorred lightning diagnoses. If a patient with advanced Parkinson's disease were to shuffle into his consulting room, Holmes would examine him minutely from head to toe and carry out searching tests for possible sensory or visual defects before ultimately deciding that the case was one of Parkinson's disease.

Understandably, Risien Russell had an enormous clientèle, for he had a quality of great elegance, and his patients felt so much better after consulting him. Lord Conway summed up this gift when, in the 17th century, he wrote to his invalid daughter: "To have a good opinion of the Physician doth contribute mutche to the care". It was believed that at Wimpole Street Risien had a suite of consulting rooms so arranged that he could see two patients at the same time. He was said to have been able to interview four patients in an hour, and that each one left his presence relieved and content. Some of his seniors looked askance at him, but not his patients who adored him, or his junior colleagues at Queen Square who thought he was marvellous.

Risien was also out of favour with most alienists, as psychiatrists were then called, and yet one of his closest friends was T.B. Hyslop, the medical superintendent of Bethlem Asylum. This unpopularity was due to his efforts to keep mildly psychotic patients out of mental institutions, where all too often they were committed for indefinite periods. Risien Russell felt strongly that injustice was often being done. He believed that many patients incarcerated in nursing homes could be perfectly well looked after by caring relations and sympathetic general practitioners. His own private practice was largely made up of psychoneurotics, to whom he gave reassurance and supportive treatment. He was a firm believer in courses of "lymphoid serum"—a precursor, perhaps, of later polyvitamin therapy.

For some years he served as Chairman of the National Society for Lunacy Reform.

Risien Russell gained notoriety and, in some quarters, unpopularity, because of the key part he played in the *cause célèbre* of the 1920s, the Harnett v. Bond case. Harnett, who had been under certificate as insane, managed to escape long enough to sue the Board of Control and also the Superintendent of the Institution for wrongful detention. He won his case and was awarded £54,000 in compensation. Sixty years ago this was an unheard-of sum within the Law Courts. The equivalent today is well over a million pounds.

While I was still his House Physician, Risien Russell remarried. His wife was a charming and gentle lady. Before this, he had entertained generously *en garçon*. He used to take me to the annual dinner of the Edinburgh ex-medical students' club in London. About twice a year he held dinner parties at his house for his neurological colleagues. As space was relatively limited, he invited the more junior doctors one evening, followed by a dinner for the seniors the next day. Dr. Greenfield, the neuropathologist who was world-famous but essentially a simple man, turned up on the wrong night, as I remember. It was a delight to see how the host immediately put the embarrassed Greenfield completely at his ease. The 10 or 12 guests sat around a huge circular table which was in the corner of the dining room. On one wall hung a beautiful painting by John Constable.

Then there were occasions when Risien held musical tea-parties at Wimpole Street. After refreshments the guests repaired to the drawing room, where chairs had been arranged and a quartet of musicians was ready to play. Once when I was invited, I can recall that Risien, for the only time in my experience, was ruffled. Two lady guests were chatting audibly while the orchestra was playing, and he was obviously offended.

He died suddenly at the age of 76, in his consulting rooms in the interval between seeing patients.

A few years before the Second World War, Sir Arthur Hurst asked me, "Why is there no biography of William Gowers? You people at Queen Square have written plenty about Hughlings Jackson, but you have ignored that other genius, Gowers". I had no explanation but promised to pursue the matter. I called on Risien Russell and suggested that he should write a biography of Gowers, for he had known him intimately. Risien was silent for a moment and then said he would seek the advice of James Taylor, who had actually been an assistant to both Jackson and to Gowers. He then asked me to come back to see him in a week's time. I did so, and Risien told me he had talked to Taylor. They had agreed not to write a biography. "Let the *Manual of Neurology* remain as his permanent memorial", he said.

The war followed, and after that there was no one left in London who had known Gowers intimately and who would have written about him. *Faute de mieux* I wrote the book myself, but wished that Risien were still alive to help me.

Today, Risien Russell is forgotten. In his time, he was one of the most important and colourful figures within the medical profession of Great Britain. He was a sincere friend and wise counsellor, and I mourn his passing.

d. 1940
Paul Schuster

This chapter is by far the most difficult I have embarked upon, largely because of lack of information. Although I repeatedly visited the clinic of Professor Paul Schuster in the years 1929–1933, and thereafter corresponded with him, the catastrophes of history intervened.

Just when and where Paul Schuster was born, I do not know, but I believe he was a Berliner. His death occurred shortly after he had made a desperate escape from Germany almost at the moment when the Second World War started. By then I was in the Royal Navy, and could not meet him. His death was merely a statistic in the Aliens' Registration files. But during those frenetic pre-Hitler days in Berlin, I realised that he was one of the greatest clinical neurologists that I had encountered. In my mind, and for the purposes of the work I was doing at that time, I bracketed him with Jean Lhermitte of Paris.

The Austro-German researches in neuro-psychiatry were considerable, and up to 1933 the German literature of this discipline was of outstanding merit. In an idiosyncratic fashion I was steadily learning the language, and was keeping well in touch with the published neurological monographs and papers in German. My various continental travels had allowed me to meet many of the great men of German neurology, some of whom became good friends of mine.

The famous Georg Schaltenbrand was the earliest in this company, and when we first met he was an assistant at the Eppendorfer Krankenhaus in Hamburg. Through him I met his chief, Pette, and also that all-powerful figure Max Nonne— then an incredibly old man. Nonne had never recovered from the loss of his son, a soldier in the first World War, and I was warned that he refused to meet British or American visitors. However, he gave me an interview, and I found him to be a courteous, kindly but frail old gentleman.

Years later, when Schaltenbrand was occupying the Chair in Würzburg, he introduced me to one of the most eccentric figures in neurology, Professor Scheller. He received me in his study in the company of two—or was it three—enormous but friendly dogs. On shelves around the room, many small stones—fragments of granite and of marble—were arranged and labelled. His hobby was to visit the burial places of notable figures in Germany and elsewhere, and to filch a stone from each grave as a memento. To Schaltenbrand I also owed the pleasure of meeting that truly delightful neuropathologist, Alois Jakob.

My many visits to the Berlin of Christopher Isherwood brought me in contact with the aloof Bonhoeffer and his assistant Thiele, and also Hirschfeld. At that time Berlin was indeed an odd city, unsettled, even sinister. The coloured lights of the Kurfürstendamm illuminated an artificial and dissolute gaiety. There was the huge, brash Kempinsky's Haus Vaterland; the restaurant Femina with its *Tischtelefonen;* and nightclubs patronised by transvestites. Berlin, never very handsome, had become a city of the plain.

But below this shoddy façade, medical science flourished. At the Charité Hospital, I also met Creutzfeldt, having previously been warned not to be put off by his uncouth manners . . . "he had been a Naval officer in the war". Certainly he greeted me sitting down, and, as he was wearing rubber gloves, presented me the tip of his elbow for me to shake. When we met again it was I who was the Naval officer and he was working in Kiel, regardless of the devastation around him. On both occasions I found him to be affable, and his manners faultless. He seemed totally preoccupied by the fatal cases of tri-chlor-ethyl-phosphate poisoning, the result of using for cooking purposes oil from the nearby torpedo factory.

Because of my interest in injuries due to lightning and to electric currents, I made it my business when I was in Berlin to call on Professor Panse, who had written a fascinating monograph on the effects of lightning. He arranged a meeting between us and von Alvensleben, an electrical engineer who had worked with Panse. In turn, they gave me a letter to Professor Jellinek, the best known figure in electropathology, who had a department at the Allgemeine Krankenhaus in Vienna given over to the care of victims of industrial electrical injuries. Years later, Professor Panse was transferred to the Rhineland. There he was asked to examine and submit a medical report upon the mass-murderer Peter Kürten, the "Monster of Düsseldorf".

In recalling this galaxy of contributors to our knowledge of the workings of the nervous system, there stands out conspicuously the figure of Otto Foerster, the learned neurologist who had been tempted to exercise his skill as a surgeon. He, at any rate, has received a measure of recognition and is unlikely, for a generation or so at any rate, to be forgotten. Elsewhere I have written of my encounters with this great man.

The magnet that drew me to Berlin again and again was Professor Paul Schuster. He was then in charge of the Hufeland Krankenhaus, a large hospital reserved for patients who were senile or else victims of some chronic neurological disorder. It was reminiscent of the Hospice Paul Brousse in Paris. Paul Schuster was a most accomplished clinician, deeply interested in his work. He possessed an enthusiasm that was infectious. Warm and most cordial in spirit, he frequently invited me to his home, where I met his wife, their son and their daughter.

In many respects, Schuster reminded me of Jean Lhermitte. Both were men of extreme erudition, and both shared my interest in out-of-the-way aspects of neurology. Whenever I brought up a topic, however bizarre or outlandish, Schuster—like Lhermitte and Kinnier Wilson—would have something pertinent and stimulating to add. At one dinner party I happened to mention my curiosity concerning the phenomenon of inspiratory speech. At once Schuster made many observations, all of which were relevant, unexpected and thought-provoking.

It was, of course, Schuster's work on the *Greifreflex* that played no little part in prompting Adie and myself to study the complicated phenomenon of forced grasping and groping.

Schuster and I also met in Berne on the occasion of the 1st International Congress of Neurology in 1931. I read a paper dealing with the syndrome of occlusion of the superior cerebellar artery. Schuster expressed great interest, for he too had collected a series of some half dozen patients who had succumbed to this disorder, autopsy confirming the diagnosis. He suggested to me that we should work together on a paper upon this subject. He would concentrate on the clinical consequences of occlusion of that vessel, and I was to deal with the anatomy of the artery. Furthermore, he said, we should read a paper on this subject at the Berlin Neurological Society. This we did on 15th March 1932; Dr. K. Loewenstein presided. I described the morphology, and Schuster followed me with the clinical aspects. The paper was discussed by Bonhoeffer and by Kramer. It was subsequently published in the *Zeitschrift. N.P.*, 1933.

Fifty years later—almost to the day—I again gave a talk to the same Society. On this occasion I think I was better understood, for I spoke in English. The Society graciously presented me with a certificate commemorating these two occasions, and made me an Honorary Member. This was one of the most considerate acts of recognition I have known.

How I wish I could dip more deeply into "the pit of my Forgot", as the Welsh say. Now I cannot even visualise Schuster's features, which perhaps indicates a poor visual memory. Only the *persona* remains, wise, gentle, friendly and, I fear, constantly anxious.

At the time I was visiting the Hufeland Hospital, there was frantic activity in German politics. Voting was taking place for the post of Chancellor, and leaflets were dropping from balloons floating over Berlin. Day after day the newspaper headlines grew bigger and bigger. At dinner one night I asked Schuster,

"Who is this chap Hitler?". Schuster testily replied, "An hysteric, and a dangerous one at that".

I detected at the Charité Hospital a certain coolness when Schuster's name was mentioned, and it has been suggested to me that it was because he was a "pure" clinical neurologist who surpassed his colleagues in that field. More likely, however, it was because Schuster was Jewish, a fact which at the time seemed wholly irrelevant to me. He had one close friend, however, in Max Bielschowsky, then working with Oskar Vogt at the Neurobiologisches Universitäts-Laboratorium at Berlin-Buch.

Schuster sent me to Bielschowsky, and I found him to be friendly but worried. He seemed to hold Vogt in a certain awe or distrust, and he was relieved because Vogt was temporarily elsewhere when I arrived. Bielschowsky showed me sections of Lenin's brain where, it was alleged, there was an inordinate development of the granular layer of the frontal cortex. This observation had been put forward at a recent medical meeting as evidence of Lenin being a kind of *Ubermensch*. Mingazzini, a volatile neurologist from Mussolini's Rome, had strongly disagreed, arguing that a six-fingered individual was not necessarily a potential pianist.

Not for many years after 1933 did I revisit Berlin, but Schuster and I kept up a correspondence. I heard with alarm that the Hufeland Hospital had been taken over by the S.A. as a barracks. It was obvious that Schuster was in peril as long as he remained in Germany, and I pleaded with him to come to England. He sent his son to London and his daughter, who was a lawyer, to Paris, but he himself obstinately remained. I tried to interest British Jewry in his plight, but nothing materialised. At that time I was honorary visiting neurologist to the London Jewish Hospital, although I am not a Jew, and I was ready to make way for Schuster to occupy that post. But in vain.

Paul Schuster and his wife eventually reached London a few weeks before war broke out in 1939, bringing with him a crate of medical books which he gave to me, although I did not see him because I was not in London at the time; his friend, Bielschowsky had preceded him. Both Schuster and Bielschowsky died within months of each other in 1940, and their ashes lie in close apposition in a London crematorium. In the war, Schuster's daughter was arrested in Paris and never heard of again.

My memories of Paul Schuster and my regret at the subsequent neglect of his work, were the catalyst for this collection of essays. Recently I had tried to retrieve his obituary notices. Only one came to light. It had appeared in the British Medical Journal, and when I read it I realised that I had been the author. There was no other mention of him that I could trace in the neurological literature.

Although an outstanding figure in German neurology, he is now completely forgotten even in the city in which he lived and worked. Of course, he was not the most distinguished figure in his speciality, and he did not occupy an important University chair. But I had been impressed to find such an erudite and enthusiastic neurologist in charge of a community of chronic and incurable patients. Apart from the Hospice Paul Brousse in Paris, this was something outside my experience. Schuster was not a resident superintendent. He was an expert with professorial status who had dedicated himself to the study of what seemed to be an unpromising and unpopular aspect of medicine. He visited his patients daily and investigated each one thoroughly. His assistants, men like Drs. Pinéas, List, Taterka, were all experienced neurologists. Though not a prolific contributor to the literature, Schuster had written papers which were all-important and stimulating. His enthusiasm and his obvious skill as a clinician working in a *terra paene incognita,* aroused my admiration and sparked off my friendship.

But Paul Schuster lived in the wrong place and at the wrong time, and posthumous ignoral seems inevitable. My meagre recollections, I hope, may do something to re-establish him within the pantheon of our discipline. Hazlitt said, "No man is truly great who is great only in his lifetime. The test of greatness is the page of history". Hazlitt was a fine essayist, but he was not omniscient. There are exceptions, and I believe Schuster was one. As the son of Sirach wrote, "Some there be that have no memorial, who are perished as though they had never been born. Such renown as they had, time has blotted out; and on them the iniquity of oblivion has blindly scattered her poppy".

Non omnis moriar.

1885–1973
Sir Francis Walshe

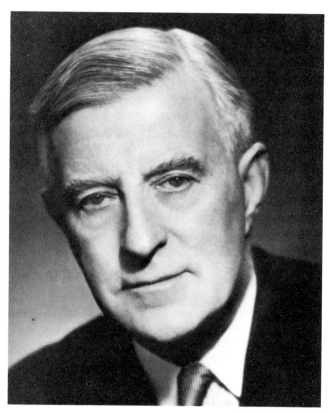

SIR FRANCIS WALSHE

nyone looking for a biography of Francis Martin Rouse Walshe, should consult the tribute written by Professor C. G. Phillips and printed in the *Biographical Memoirs of Fellows of The Royal Society*, Volume 20, December 1974. An account of Dr. Walshe's career and accomplishments is set out there in detail and with a rare discrimination.

For a period of 50 years Walshe was my mentor and close friend, but I do not find it easy to do justice to my recollections of this inimitable and peerless man who was, in many ways, unique. My memories are not a series of isolated incidents, but rather a continuing reminiscence spanning half a century.

For sheer intellectualism he towered above his colleagues, highly gifted individualists though they were. But he was a nullifidian; one who could detect with uncanny sagacity the flaws or weak points in a proposition or a theory. It is because he was largely regarded as a critic, that I fear he may be forgotten in years to come. His barbed disparagements offended many, for there was no one like Walshe when it came to distinguishing hocus from pocus. As if his role as a derogator were not enough, he laced his comments with a devastating wit. As Prime Minister Bonar Law said of Lord Birkenhead, "It would be easier for him to keep a live coal in his mouth than a witty saying". Walshe knew well that he possessed this idiosyncrasy, and sometimes asserted that he regretted the fact. I doubt this, for he had such a glorious sense of fun—rare in a wit—that he thoroughly enjoyed each quip.

But while criticism may be refuted, not so a jest. Hence the combination of banter with rebuke was apt to prove humiliating to some who had felt the sharp edge of his tongue. Many scientists whose researches had been criticised by Walshe, bore a lifelong resentment. However, some of his more forgiving victims ended up by falling under his spell.

On my arrival in Queen Square in 1923, I was allotted to Walshe as his House Physician. He had then been on the consulting staff for a couple of years, having served an unusually long stint as Resident Medical Officer before the 1914–1918 war. Walshe was also a member of the recently formed Medical Unit at University College Hospital. He was born in London, his father being an Irishman from County Mayo and his mother a Devonian from Brixham. One of his paternal ancestors had been hanged after the 1798 rebellion. Walshe was thus in good company, for a similar fate befell two of Hughlings Jackson's ancestors captured after the Battle of Sedgemoor in 1685.

In 1923 Walshe was carrying out clinical researches based on physiological principles. He was able to show, by temporarily deafferenting various muscle-groups in patients with Parkinson's disease, a reduction in rigidity but no influence upon tremor.

Walshe was greatly impressed by the experimental work in animals on tonic neck reflexes carried out in the Netherlands by Magnus and De Kleijn. He demonstrated that these phenomena could be elicited in man, especially when a hemiplegia was present; also when there was a spastic paraparesis suggestive of the decerebrate rigidity observed in the laboratory. The elicitation of the Babinski response in the great toe was, Walshe found, liable to qualitative alterations according to such factors as turning of the head to one side; changes in the posture of the trunk and lower limbs; and also the injection of hyoscine.

Already Walshe had begun his career as a forceful critic. His difference of opinion with Professor Gowland Hopkins was still smouldering. Gowland Hopkins, the discoverer of vitamins, considered that peripheral neuritis was a deficiency disorder. Walshe believed there also existed in the aetiology, a toxic factor.

A fresh target for attack came up in Australia, when Hunter

and Royle hypothesized a control of striped muscle exercised by the autonomic nervous system. Although this idea received some measure of support from his colleague in anatomy, Grafton Elliot Smith, the notion did not stand up to scrutiny and was soon forgotten, largely because of Walshe's critical reviews.

As we went through the wards, Walshe gave the impression of being somewhat remote. Perhaps it would be more true to say that he seemed preoccupied. This attitude soon melted, for he formed the habit of joining me in my sitting room in the hospital, where he relaxed and chatted freely. This was neurological gossip at its best, and his comments upon the contemporary scene, including many of his colleagues, were often somewhat captious and indiscreet. Nonetheless, he had his heroes—Gordon Holmes, Sherrington, Magnus and his co-workers, the late William Gowers, and especially Hughlings Jackson and Victor Horsley. Later he developed a great admiration for Polyani and, in the United States, Lashley, Walter Riese; later still, Hans Reese. The contemporary school of French neurology he held in high regard. He was warm in his appreciation of the Toronto team of neurologists, but this came later.

In 1924, Walshe left the Medical Unit to become a consulting neurologist to University College Hospital. This move necessitated his embarking upon a private practice, which he continued until his late seventies. Otherwise his free time was devoted to writing, for he did not seem to have any hobbies or alternative forms of recreation.

Walshe might conceivably have devoted himself to academic physiology had he not—as he admitted to me—been unable to stomach the thought of a life-time spent in animal experimentation. His humane instincts drew him to become a practising physician, one who sought to help rather than to hurt.

He was surely the most handsome member of the staff at Queen Square. Tall, slim, with close-shaven clean-cut features, he dressed well, though not in the mode of Risien Russell, the local Beau Brummel. As is not uncommon, his good looks became more evident as he aged; the smooth, unimpassioned face of youth became etched with the lines traced by character and experience. Is it not said that by the age of 45 one gets the face one deserves? His hair turned gray then white but remained thick; his pallor was matched by his light gray suits. He appeared, indeed, a veritable *éminence grise,* but with a twinkle.

It did not take me long to realise that Walshe was a man of outstanding intellect. Some of his colleagues deplored that he was essentially an iconoclast, and that he had never carried out any productive research, clinical or otherwise. Actually, during the first World War, Walshe, as neurologist to the Army in Egypt, was engaged in important studies upon local epidemics of polyneuritis, beri-beri, and a common diphtheritic infection of wounds. On the whole, however, Walshe's long professional life was largely devoted to critical appraisals of the work of others. In so doing, he occupied a highly important role, and was probably the solitary individual to play such a part in medicine at any time in its recent history.

As a neurologist, he did not excel as a clinical diagnostician; nor as a lecturer; nor when giving clinical demonstrations. His supreme abilities lay in his writings, particularly those of a critical character. His command of language was superb, but he did not allow persiflage to debase the seriousness of his work. He kept his quips and wisecracks for his conversation and his letter-writing. Critics, however much disliked, occupy a vital role in medicine just as in art and science. Carlyle well said that criticism stands like an interpreter between the inspired and the uninspired. Without the critical overseer, the world would be in chaos.

After his clinico-physiological researches, Walshe dedicated himself to his role as a *malleus malificorum.* It is not that his mind was closed to new ideas. He received them, warily, and then analysed them with uncanny skill. He would unerringly detect the fallacies in the argument; the Achilles heel would become all too evident. He was never influenced by the personality or the prestige of the writer.

He launched an attack upon the parcellation of the cerebral cortex, especially Brodmann's elaborate mapping—a notion which never became popular in Great Britain.

Then came his trenchant attack upon Henry Head's concept of protopathic-epicritic sensation. Walshe was not the first to discredit the notion of a two-stage hierarchy of peripheral sensation, one older and cruder, the other younger and more discriminative. Nevertheless, Head's hypothesis lingered in neurological teaching. Walshe's *coup de grace* was delivered in 1942 when he wrote concerning the hypothetical "protopathic animal" thought up by Head and his co-worker, the psychologist Rivers. "Such a creature, even if it could take the steps necessary to propagate its bewildered kind, which appears doubtful, could have no survival value, for on receipt of a stimulus which it could not localise, from a stimulating agent whose nature it had no means of discovering, it could respond only by curling up and micturating. Yet this is the animal that Head and Rivers present to us as our common ancestor".

In the years 1947–1949 in Great Britain and elsewhere, outbreaks of poliomyelitis were common with a considerable mortality and a risk of permanent crippledom, but without means of prevention or cure or knowledge of modes of propagation. Walshe disagreed with his colleague, James Collier, on the question of what steps should be taken if an acute case cropped up in a boarding school. A spirited correspondence took place in the medical press. Collier advised that if a child in a boarding school developed polio, the other boys and girls should remain upon the premises. Walshe considered it safer for the parents to remove their unaffected children.

Even greater disapproval was displayed by Walshe against a lady doctor in Australia who advocated injections of convalescent serum in patients with acute poliomyelitis. And when Sister Kenny of Australia visited London promoting her strong views on the management of victims of acute poliomyelitis, Walshe was goaded to assert that there was something about poliomyelitis that brought out the worst in Australian womanhood.

There was also the brouhaha about the pathogenesis of multiple sclerosis. Earlier in the century, a Continental author claimed he had found in the cerebrospinal fluid of patients with this disease, spirochaetes, which he regarded as being of causal significance. The finding provoked mild interest for a while, but not for long. However, it was resuscitated when a pathologist in Glasgow also declared that he had detected in the spinal fluid, spirochaetes which were either fully formed or fragmented. Attention was aroused and much scepticism. Walshe remarked that in Scotland, microscopy had revealed something that looked like Harry Lauder's walking-stick and that this was probably the end of the story.

The claims of a spirochaetal origin were soon forgotten when Purves Stewart, neurologist to the Westminster Hospital, came on the scene. One of his biotechnical assistants, he asserted, had observed specific bodies in the spinal fluid in cases of multiple sclerosis. They spoke of a "spherula insularis", and Purves Stewart hastened to have a vaccine prepared which was used as a treatment for his patients with multiple sclerosis. This was the occasion when Walshe wrote his famous letter to a medical journal claiming that he, too, had seen a unicorn strolling in the Broad Sanctuary (that is, the area in London where the Westminster Hospital was sited). Later, the claims for a "spherula insularis" were thoroughly investigated by the Medical Research Council, and devastatingly rejected.

Walshe now directed himself towards greater targets. In a long correspondence he argued with John Fulton of Yale over the precise definition of the prefrontal cortex. Fulton, a victim of chronic ill-health, was easy-going, and no rancour developed between the two contenders. The same could not be said about Walshe's quarrels with Wilder Penfield. The latter had postulated an anatomical representation of the body within the preRolandic gyrus. He visualized a grotesque figure with a large head and prominent lips and tongue, a huge hand with a conspicuous thumb and forefinger, and a small body and legs. This was Penfield's "homunculus", but to Walshe, mindful of Alice in Wonderland, it was pure jabberwocky. Some of Walshe's strictures concerning Penfield were personal and scarcely kind. To quote Professor Phillips: "Walshe probably felt it was the critic's business to hack away the over-exuberant brushwood from the neurological jungle; his admirers saw it crackling briskly in the bright flame of his prose". Walshe was indeed "a writer, a biter and a fighter", as Hilaire Belloc said.

In addition to his serious criticisms in neurological journals, he wrote frequently to the medical Press on a variety of topics. One of his letters contradicted claims which had been made by doctors who believed in the existence of hysterical fever. Psychogenic headache also came in for attack. He believed that the "headache" complained of by hysterics was not "pain" at all but possibly some other sensory modality, the patient so afflicted remaining "as rosy as an apple and as plump as a partridge".

On a lighter note, one letter deplored the undue fouling by dogs of the pavements within the Harley Street area. He conceded that the Borough Council had attached notices to the lamp-posts threatening a fine of £5, but, wrote Walshe, the notices were "too high for the average dog to read". He signed the letter Agag (need it be pointed out that Agag was the man in the Bible who proceeded delicately).

Walshe was a Roman Catholic, but on occasions he must have been a veritable thorn in the flesh of his co-religionists. In various issues of the *Catholic Medical Guardian,* he inveighed against the claims for miraculous cures at Lourdes and elsewhere, and the belief in the stigmata of the saints. He was highly critical of the Jesuits in their role as schoolteachers.

The upsurge of interest by physiologists in the electrical activity of cerebral function, was, to Walshe, something that had got out of hand. He castigated them as belonging to the Peter Pan school of science with its "bloodless dance of action potentials" and "its hurrying to and fro of its molecules".

For years Walshe had derided those who wrote student textbooks. His attitude may have originated when the comparatively young Russell Brain—the "neurological Messiah", as Walshe called him—published a *Manual of Nervous Disorders.* Imagine our surprise, therefore, when there appeared in 1940 a slim *Textbook of Nervous Diseases* by F.M.R. Walshe. He hastened to assure us that his little book was something different, in that it was made up of nothing but simple fundamental facts devoid of hypotheses and speculations. His book became popular and ran into eleven editions in 30 years. Had he lived longer, there would no doubt have been more. He had become quite fond of his *Child's Guide to Neurology,* as he called it.

When first published, it was passed for review to Dr. Robert Wartenberg, that nit-picker of literature who had already become unpopular because of his scathing criticisms of some highly respected American textbooks. Wartenberg was uneasy about going into print with adverse comments on something Walshe had written. He felt it behoved him to write to Walshe and explain how reluctant he had been to take issue with a master whom he held in the greatest regard, and so on. Walshe's reply—written *en clair* on a postcard—was laconic. "Don't be a silly ass. Yours, F.M.R.W."

In 1952 we travelled to North America together. On 8th May we embarked in the Ile de France. At dinner that night we were presented with a menu the size of a newspaper. At the bottom was a note stating that invalids on special diets were catered for. We summoned the Head Steward, and I told him that my companion suffered from a caviare-deficiency. "Yes", murmured Walshe, "severe chronic asturgeonosis". No more was said, but thereafter we were offered caviare with every meal.

We separated temporarily in New York, I to stay in Dr. David Ross's apartment in Irving Place, and Walshe in the Commodore Hotel. A couple of days later, I called on him. He was seated in the lobby alongside a Catholic priest. Walshe remarked to him, "Wasn't it Shelley who said that hell is a city very like

London? Father, Shelley had never been to New York". Walshe told me that he had that afternoon lectured to the students at Columbia. "I told them they must not think that physiology began with the introduction of electroencephalography; it didn't, any more than civilisation began with the Declaration of Independence". When I enquired as to the effect of his oratory, he said that for about 20 seconds there was a deadly silence during which you could hear their neurological pins dropping, and then there was a roar of laughter.

We dined at the house of Harold Alsop Riley, finding ourselves in the genial company of the Houston Merritts, Sam Wortis, Mrs. Foster Kennedy and Harold Wolff. It was a perfect party and Walshe made a big impression on the others, who obviously enjoyed his conversation.

Walshe proceeded to Harvard, where he lectured. Afterwards an astonished Bostonian remarked to him, "With that name of yours and your gift of the gab, you could have been Governor of Massachusetts".

There was an occasion when Walshe was invited to Baltimore to consider accepting a professorial appointment at Johns Hopkins Hospital. He enjoyed his visit immensely, but decided he did not want to leave London. He told me of some extraordinary cases he had seen there. One was a man who had been caught *in flagrante delicto* with his neighbour's wife. The husband drew his gun and shot the patient through the spine. The bullet lodged in the conus medullaris, with the clinical result that the victim was rendered doubly incontinent and impotent. Walshe said he did not know which to admire the more, the husband's knowledge of anatomy or his marksmanship.

Like most clinical neurologists, Walshe did some medico-legal work. His appearances in the Law Courts were memorable. Cross-examining Counsel were fair game for Walshe's repartee. In one compensation case, the opposing medical witness made some statements which Walshe regarded as preposterous, irrelevant and completely different from his own views. When Counsel expostulated, "But, Dr. Walshe, do you not support the opinion of our distinguished expert?", Walshe replied, "What your witness had to say was like the flowers that bloom in the Spring, tra-la" (that is, nothing to do with the case!).

On another occasion he gave evidence for the plaintiff, a 19-year-old girl with a severe post-traumatic syndrome. The cross-examining Counsel said, "You will agree, Dr. Walshe, that the outlook is likely to be relatively favourable in a healthy young adult?". Walshe replied, "If you wish me to say that 19 is the ideal age for a fractured skull, I cannot agree. I would say 99".

Every neurologist of that era had his own "Walshism" to narrate and to chuckle over, or sometimes to deprecate. Professor Phillips rightly deemed them inappropriate for inclusion within his official biography. But I quote one here as exemplifying the brilliant and engaging man I so admired. Once when Walshe was presiding over a medical congress, I was the Secretary and there were just the two of us on the daïs. The speaker was a lady doctor named Helen. Suddenly Walshe whispered in my ear, enquiring whether I could tell him the unit of female beauty. On my expressing ignorance, Walshe said, "One micro-Helen; that is, the face that launched *one* ship". Recently I was amused to hear this quip on the radio, 38 years later, but it was attributed to a living source. I have no reason to believe that it was not an original remark of Walshe's.

Although he occasionally attended race-meetings, as far as I could determine, Walshe had no hobbies other than writing. In addition to his important contributions to *Brain* and his letters to the medical Press, Walshe carried on a large correspondence with friends—and, indeed, anyone with whom he wanted to take issue whether or not he knew them. Dr. McNaughten of Montreal asserted that a collection of Walshe's letters would be a publisher's dream.

Even through his 8th and 9th decades, his mind was fecund and he continued to write. He readily accepted invitations to contribute to journals with which I was concerned. Robert Frost expressed well this *cacoëthes scribendi:*

The words are lovely, dark and deep
But I have promises to keep
And miles to go before I sleep
And miles to go before I sleep.

Walshe was elected in 1946 to the Fellowship of the Royal Society; a distinction rarely accorded to a practising clinician. Further recognition came rather belatedly in the form of a knighthood. Walshe cynically observed to me that if he had been a jockey he would have been honoured years earlier.

How many neurologists are now aware of the opposition which Walshe entertained towards the inception of the National Health Service? It was not that he objected to the principle of medical care being made available gratuitously, but he resented the idea of hospitals being State-funded, and the consultants no longer being "honoraries" but paid officials. Still more, he disliked the concept of "merit" awards. Walshe therefore carried out his hospital practice faithfully, but he refused to accept any payment whatsoever for his services.

When Walshe reached the statutory retirement age of 65, the Chairman of the National Hospital, Sir Ernest Gowers (son of the great William Gowers), ordained that Walshe's period of service should be extended to the age of 70. The Medical Committee concurred, but the vote was far from unanimous and an understanding was reached that never again would such an extension be granted. Earlier, Hughlings Jackson had been allowed to stay on the staff until the age of 75.

Of necessity, Walshe continued in private practice long after he was 70. I and one or two other colleagues took some of his patients into beds on our service, and when he gave up his consulting rooms he carried on his practice in a room of mine in Queen Square.

The matter of retirement was raised jokingly between us from time to time. We debated what we should do with ourselves when we were too old to see patients. The fact that there was a 15-year age-gap between us did not arise. One idea we entertained—not too seriously, I hasten to say—was for us to open a pub near Harley Street, preferably not too far from the premises of the General Medical Council. We could thereby count on customers who wished to celebrate their reprieve from the Disciplinary Committee, as well as those who sought to drown their sorrows. We could not agree, however, on the name of our pub. It was to be either "The Up-Going Toe" or "Charcot's Joint".

Eventually Walshe decided, reluctantly, that the time had come for him to leave London, and to live quietly in the country. To his surprise and delight, he found considerable enjoyment in a Huntingdonshire village in his pretty little house with its walled garden and a stream. He would make a weekly visit to London to see patients or to attend a dinner, but gradually he gave up doing so and devoted himself to reading and writing. From time to time I would visit him. He had been a patient of mine for a few years. By his 87th year his health deteriorated and he died at the age of 88, mourned by the dwindling number of those who had known him well.

Shortly afterwards I had the privilege of giving the eulogy at a service of thanksgiving for his life and work which was held in the chapel of the National Hospital. I ended it, as I do now, with Chaucer's words:

He loved chivalrye,
Trouthe and honour, freedom and curteisye,
He was a verray parfit gentil Knight.

1886–1962
Israel Wechsler

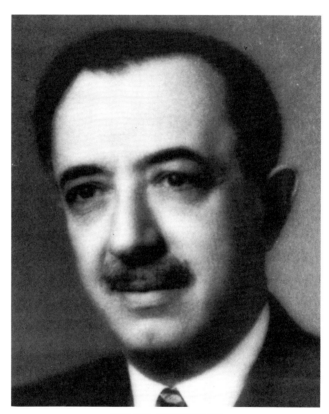

ISRAEL WECHSLER

Courtesy of the Journal of the Mount Sinai Hospital, New York.

My meeting with this distinguished and good man was an indirect outcome of World War II. One of the team of neuropsychiatric specialists organised by me and Professor Desmond Curran was Surgeon Lieutenant-Commander David Ross. When the war ended, this officer was offered a civil appointment in the U.S.A., and early in the 1950s he was established as Resident Medical Director of a hospital for speech disorders in Irving Place, Manhattan. When I visited North America in 1952, I stayed with him in New York.

David Ross also invited me to lecture at his hospital, and I spoke about some aspect of speech or language. My audience was a distinguished one, and included Dr. Eisenson (Palo Alto), Dr. Levin (of the Kleine-Levin syndrome), Professor Kurt Goldstein and also Israel Wechsler, then Chief of Neurology at Mount Sinai Hospital. Goldstein and Wechsler took me off to dinner with them afterwards. I did not record in my diary the name of the restaurant, but, unless there is a considerable hole in my memory, it was Luchow's.

Over the ensuing years, Wechsler and I often met. Sometimes we were in the company of Morris Bender, sometimes Kurt Goldstein. Once, Israel Wechsler invited his famous psychologist brother, David, to join us. On another occasion, he motored Bender, Diamond and me from Atlantic City to New York, and I spent the night in his apartment.

Israel Wechsler was a high-spirited companion, for he was witty and was endowed with a great sense of the ridiculous. He was a gifted and amusing raconteur, and an entertaining conversationalist. "I can only remember the pattern and weight of these conversations, not the substance", as Lawrence Durrell said. In addition, he was a man of wide culture who was fluent in many tongues, including French, German, Hebrew, Yiddish and, presumably, Rumanian. His knowledge of Shakespeare was quite exceptional, and apparently he was vastly erudite in the history and theology of Judaism. He was a fervent Zionist, and was Chairman of the Friends of the Hebrew University whence he received an honorary doctorate of philosophy. The Hebrew University also dignified him by establishing an Israel Wechsler Chair in Neurology. He had written a scholarly monograph upon Moses ben Maimon, better known as Maimonides.

It became obvious that Wechsler had many friends among the writers, scientists and poets in New York. He often spoke to me of Einstein.

I was particularly interested to learn that he was born and brought up in Rumania, leaving at the age of 14 for the U.S.A. and knowing no English at the time. Once, for three weeks, I had been Visiting Professor to Bucharest, a city that had been called the Paris of Eastern Europe. It was an interesting assignment, for I learned to appreciate the manner in which they were keeping alive the memory of their best-known neurologist, Marinesco. I left Rumania with warm memories of their neurology and neurosurgery, their gerontological researches, their hospitality, the beauty of Sinaia, the summer resort, and, above all, their music. In the past, Rumanian neurology had been chiefly allied to the Charcot school, and it was, therefore, a pleasure to meet a Rumanian neurologist established in New York.

It is a matter of great regret to me that I did not see more of this charming and cultivated man. In particular, I did not have the opportunity of attending his clinic and watching him at work.

In 1956, it was my privilege to welcome Wechsler to the National Hospital, where he delivered a most interesting address. In introducing him to the audience, I told them—with his permission and to his enjoyment—a tale which was no doubt apochryphal. His secretary in New York once answered the telephone and heard a middle-European voice asking whether she was speaking to Dr. Wechsler's office. Told that she was, the voice went on, "Is he the neurologist?". "Uh, uh". "Say, does he also see psychiatric patients?". "Uh, uh". "What's his fee?". She was told. There was a pause and then "Crazy that much, I am not. Goodbye."

Wechsler certainly welcomed patients with psychiatric and neurotic disorders. He was, indeed, a true neuropsychiatrist. He had paid long visits to Freud in Vienna, but he was no psycho-analyst. He believed profoundly in Freud's conception of the unconscious, but he was hostile to the idea of psycho-analysis as a form of therapy.

His literary output was considerable and its quality was high, containing many original concepts and ideas. He enjoyed teaching, an art in which he excelled. In 1927 Wechsler wrote a textbook of clinical neurology, which achieved popularity and ran into nine editions in his lifetime. A volume of essays appeared in 1950 under the title *The Neurologist's Point of View*. Among the papers were articles upon "The History of Neurology", "The History of Psychiatry", "Racial Psychology", "Anti-Semitism", "A Critical Appreciation of Sigmund Freud", "Palestinian and Russian Colonization".

Although these essays were written four decades ago they are still readable, being clear and well argued. More than that, they were written with elegance. He dedicated his collection of essays to a medical student of great promise, "To the memory of my son, Robert Moses, the best friend I ever had".

Even in his lifetime an Israel Wechsler lectureship was established, and I was honoured by an invitation to deliver one of these addresses, on 9th December 1960.

Death came in 1962 in his 76th year. His colleague, Professor Nachmansohn, spoke feelingly of him as a dynamic and colourful individual whose passing was a personal loss to numerous friends, causing many gaps, but whose creative achievements had erected a monument that would continue to live.

In Gulliver's Laputa, men of honour, justice, wisdom and learning were exempt from all forms of taxation. Had this favour existed in Manhattan, Israel Wechsler would have been one of the first to qualify.

Epilogue

These were all my friends. There were many others, some eminent others not, but for various reasons they do not belong here.

I have outlived them and my recollections have survived. Writing these essays has been my personal memorial to them. What I have written "has been begot in the ventricle of memory, nourished in the womb of *pia mater,* and delivered upon the mellowing of occasion" (*"Love's Labour's Lost",* William Shakespeare*).*

* * * * * *

But you have gone now, all of you, that were so beautiful when quick with life. Yet not gone, for you are still a living truth inside my mind. So how are you dead . . . when you live with me as surely as I live myself.

Shall we say that good Dr. Johnson is dead, when his dear friend Mr. Boswell brings him to thunder and thump before your very eyes? Is Socrates dead, then, when I hear the gold of his voice?

Are my friends all dead, then, and their voices a glory in my ears?

No, and I will stand to say no, and no, again.
How Green Was My Valley, Richard Llewellyn.